Separated From The Light:

A Path Back From Psychological Trauma

Second Edition

By:
William B. Tollefson, Ph.D.

TOLLEFSON ENTERPRISES

Cape Coral, Florida

© Copyright 1997

Inner Values Incorporated / Tollefson

All rights reserved. No part of this publication may be reproduced or transmitted in any form or by any means, electronic or mechanical, including photocopy. No recording or any other information storage and/or retrieval system without permission in writing from Inner Values Incorporated.

Published by Tollefson Enterprises

Second Edition 2004

First Edition August 1997

ISBN 0-9760554-0-6

Printed in the United States of America

10 9 8 7 6 5 4 3 2 1

To learn more about the
Women's Institute for Incorporation Therapy:
www.wiit.com
E-Mail: recovery@wiit.com
(800) 437-5478

Separated From The Light

"The windows to ourselves are sometimes clouded by the winds of terror and frosted by the chill of loyalty, therefore our darkness continues."

William Tollefson

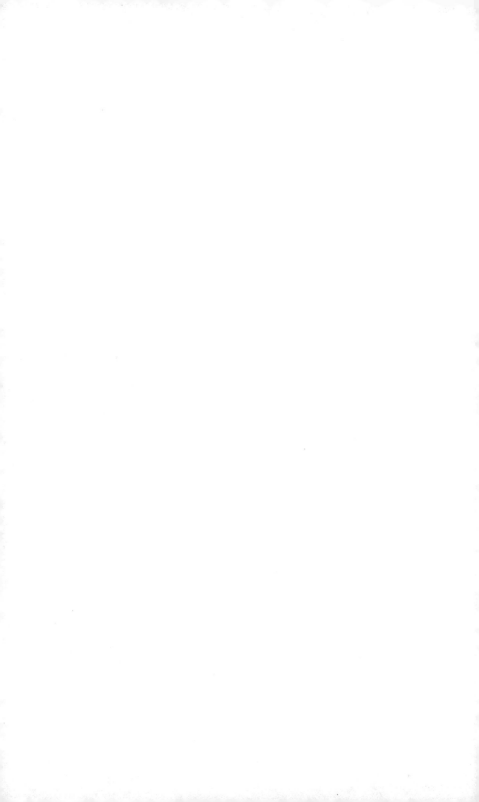

Dedicated in memory of
William G. and Barbara Ann Tollefson

I am particularly grateful to my wife Melody and my daughter Tammi Ann,
for their loving support and inspiration.

I'm also very grateful to Leslie Ann Kent
and Tammy Burton.

My thanks to Julia Lee Dulfer for her wonderful
work in editing this book.

Thanks to my partner Larry Spinosa and his wife Diane
for their extensive efforts on this manuscript.

Without all of their help this book would not
have been possible.

Table of Content

Introduction 3

Part I

Chapter 1 Living Nightmare 7
Chapter 2 Pain 25
Chapter 3 Discovery 37
Chapter 4 Inner Journey 69

Part II

Chapter 5 "What Do I Need to Change?" 101
Chapter 6 The Unfolding Self 113
Chapter 7 Recovery 143
Chapter 8 Incorporation Therapy 165
Chapter 9 Steps Toward Recovery 173
Epilogue 177
Bibliography 179

Separated from the Light

Introduction

This book was written to let people know that there is effective help for Post-Traumatic Stress Disorder (PTSD), and there are professionals who can assist with their recovery. It offers common-sense principles and theory explaining what a human being does in reaction to trauma and suggests a possible path to recovery. *Separated from the Light* illuminates the darkness, isolation, and secrecy that shroud survivors of trauma. It celebrates the power, strength, intelligence, and creativity that all survivors demonstrate in their pursuit of self-preservation in the face of danger. It brings a perception of normalcy to the survival process and helps survivors understand the commonality of their reactions.

Separated from the Light presents two views of the mental, physical, emotional and/or spiritual, post effects of trauma: 1) The survivor's perspective, 2) the educational view of the mechanics involved in what I term the symbolic unfolding process.

Some people conceptualize life events better through experiencing stories, and others understand better by thinking through a process. This book offers both. The first half is fuel for the heart and the second is fuel for the mind. If the reader empathizes with the character in the clinical story, then their ability to understand the mechanics will be enhanced. Part two is a mirror image of part one.

Since the dawn of human civilization, storytelling has been used to impart information by way of the spoken word, symbolic pictures, or later the written word. It's a powerful method of passing down knowledge of the strength and power that we human beings possess. It is a safe way of addressing the deep symbolism present in trauma and the process of surviving those experiences.

Part one gives the reader a chance to identify with the internal reaction to trauma, i.e., the loss of self. The story offers a glimpse into the survivor's emotional struggle and the mental battlefield on which it is fought, even when that battle occurs years after the traumatic event. The tale is a composite of clinical information from many survivors. The telling of this story is a simple means of understanding the hidden world of pain and horror. It gives the reader a way to see from the inside out the intrusive and repetitive suffering that is common among survivors.

Part two examines the same issues but from an educational perspective. It offers a look at the creative mechanics of the loss-of-self process that is enacted for survival. This part of the book is a common-sense approach to my basic theory and stated principles of how a person symbolically unfolds to save self in reaction to a traumatic invasion by an overwhelming force. It will assist the reader in understanding that a person doesn't break when overwhelmed by trauma. Rather, the victim unfolds as miraculously as a butterfly emerging from its chrysalis and takes flight to safety.

I believe that those who survive a trauma do so because of their strength, intelligence, power, and creativity. It is my belief that any who survive horrifying events do so through interaction between mind, body, and spirit – elements working in unity to hide "self" safely away in a maze of dissociative symbols. I believe such internal interaction is a gift from God (or higher power) and is an ability present from birth. This phenomenon is an instinctive and natural restructuring of the mind, body, spirit, and self. It's a miracle that protects a person from any outside agent, natural or human, that attempts to strip control of self from them through force.

Self doesn't disappear; it hides deep within but doesn't remain quiet forever. Self acts out in anger, crying for attention gained by releasing damaging thoughts, feelings, or behaviors. It speaks in "disguised communication" using symbolic messages. Yet its meaning is clear, self yearns to be rescued.

Knowledge acquired about the daunting symptoms of trauma diminishes their power and mystery. Wisdom gained from reading *Separated from the Light* should shine into the darkness of trauma survivors, thereby empowering self and reducing the fear and anxiety associated with past events.

William B. Tollefson, Ph.D

Part One

Chapter 1

Living Nightmare

    The thought popped into her head as she sat in the front passenger seat of a 1999 gun metal gray Ford Explorer. It arose between the pain of the reality that she was en route to a mental hospital and the intense need to escape. If she had read that line in a book it would have made her chuckle. She stared past the dew-misted glass of the car window, trying not to make a sound when the emotional pains came, hoping not to alert the driver. She tried not to think about her second husband, David, tried not to think about anything. But sometimes the thoughts just came up. Tall, muscular-framed David standing there in his military fatigues right in front of her, fire in his eyes, one hand with a beer in it, and the other a semi-clenched fist used to slap her. She kind of wished he was there. She would have enjoyed seeing "Mr. Control" realize he had been fooled.

    She began rolling down the window, and the dampness of the inrushing air hit Barbara Ann Freeman's sullen face. She recognized a slight increase in her heart rate. The coming night began to heighten her awareness. Barbara's thoughts were drawn from the present into fear of what her future would bring. Darkness always brought on haunting feelings in the recesses of her mind. The secrets she had unknowingly guarded all these years no longer remained quiet within her. Barb, as she liked to be called, knew that nighttime would plunge her back into the depths of a world of fragmented images and threatening sounds.

    During the past six months Barb's repressed memories refused to stay dormant. Memories of her early childhood lay quietly in the shadows of her mind, remaining hidden for her protection. She could only recall the years since her eleventh birthday. Like a drinking glass shattered on the kitchen floor, the primary stages of Barb's life were broken into many fragments of grotesque images that kept her suspended in unbearable pain.

The crawling pressure continued to mount in the center of her head and was working its way toward the base of her neck. She felt her vigilance take over. Suddenly she was frightened by a disturbance in the air around her, directing her attention inward.

Barb's mind reflected on her past and how she had always given up control to someone else allowing others to direct and validate her feelings, thoughts, and behaviors. She never did much of anything for fear of making a mistake. She didn't want the pain of being wrong, but she always seemed to be wrong. Without someone directing her, she was left to her own internal control that she couldn't trust. Black emptiness crept into her life whenever she attempted to assert herself. As long as she could remember, other people's ideas and opinions were more important than hers, particularly her father's. She was totally unaware of where she had learned such thoughts and feelings.

Growing up, Barb idolized her father. She constantly vied with other people for his attention, even with her own family members. Yet she harbored resentment against him deep in the core of her soul. She had no idea from where those contaminated thoughts erupted. Intense fear, rage, and love surfaced whenever she thought of him. Barb never examined her incongruent feelings. He had always professed his love for her and spoken of her as his favorite in front of others, including her brothers and sisters. While he was the same man she thought she loved, he was the very person who hurt and terrorized her and she had been defending him throughout her life.

Barb's mother, on the other hand, brought on repeated waves of anger, betrayal, and competition. She was driven to please her mother, but nothing she did was good enough. She felt as though she were a threat to her mother's happiness. Funny as it may sound, she also felt she was a threat to her mother's marriage. Despite years of brutal criticism and physical mistreatment by her mother, Barb continued trying to win her love and approval. How could I have ruined that lady's life? Barb pondered. Confusion set in, stifling her racing thoughts for a moment.

A painful chain of thought formed in her mind like the dark wall of a storm. Panic coursed through her body. She frantically searched for a behavior that would numb the pain. A surge of anguish forced her to recollect fragments of foggy images. She began to see the years she consumed alcohol and drugs, the toll her addictive behavior took on her relationships, her body, her life, and her dreams.

A window that her mind blacked out years ago opened, releasing painful images of her first marriage to Steven. He was a self-made success in the construction business but troubled and haunted by his own past. Five years of torturous images raced through her brain. At last Barb analyzed why she took all that punishment, constantly living in a state of fear and guarding against Steven's next outburst. She chuckled silently at the distorted excuses she thought up. She had protected him and his career just the way she had her father's. Her rueful laughter stopped in a rush of sadness. From the pain Steven inflicted she had developed disgust for her physical self and concluded it was her body that attracted Steven's brutal attacks.

Rotating her head slowly toward the car window, Barb gazed out in an attempt to distract her thoughts and building emotions. She sought relief by forcing her mind to escape into the dark on the other side of the glass, certain the sanctuary of numbness lay less than a windowpane's thickness away.

Another onslaught of latent emotion swept over her. Barb had been battered by such upsurges for months; but if the truth were told, she had known similar episodes her whole life. The emotional attacks were taking a toll on her body and mind, and this last one almost depleted her reserves. Exhausted, she focused on the passing gray shadows of the night, hoping the scenery would dissipate her pain. But it held.

Barb finally achieved success, and passage into her sanctuary was granted. It was a magical world she entered, a safe haven from her distress. As a child she had created that world in the far reaches of her mind. It was a place where she could hide from her fears and reduce elevating anxiety, a protective territory that offered a reprieve from reality. Barb allowed no one on earth even the smallest glimpse of her private world. No one ever realized when she retreated to it. She even fooled her father. He never discovered her ability to leave mentally. He thought he always had total control of her body, mind, and spirit. As a result of his continuous brutal physical attacks over eighteen years, she became highly proficient at entering and exiting that world. Sometimes she even fooled herself.

Startled, Barb questioned whether her best friend and driver of the car was aware of her "zoning out" as she described it. She readied a couple of excuses in case Sandy discovered what was going on. She always had a repertoire of excuses to explain away her weird behavior. Assured that Sandy was unaware of the raging battle taking place inside her, Barb returned to the activity in her mind.

No one could ever understand our need to travel into my magical world except Annie, she thought. Annie was her dark side. Annie was created out of necessity. She served as a normal internal reaction to living in a very dysfunctional environment while she was growing up. Annie functioned as an unseen bad twin. She was Barb's made-up double of what her father called her "defective traits" (anger, intelligence, beauty, rebellion, adventurousness, emotions). Annie always got her in trouble. Just thinking was a sin by her father's standards. Both father and her mother refused to allow Barb to show any anger. She learned the hard way to not bare her anger, period. She was taught very young, "if I ever see anger on your face, I'll give you something to be angry about, and I'll make sure you never show it again." Barb birthed Annie as a defensive reaction at age four, the night when her father locked her in a closet for over twelve hours to teach her a "valuable lesson" as he described it. He left her there tied to a hook on the back of the door. Barb remembered thinking that she would die if she remained alone in there much longer. Annie developed to keep her company, to help her through the pain, and to give her support in the cold darkness of the closet. Barb knew she had been the compliant daughter, the "good girl" as her father put it, but Annie never knuckled under to him or to either of her husbands. She was Barb's historian, whose original function was to witness and record the endless successions of traumas so Barb didn't have to be present or feel overwhelming pain or emotions. She then stored the records far from Barb's knowledge.

At one point in her young adult life Barb thought she was one of those crazy women she had seen on television professing to have other people inside them. Wondering if she was a plain crazy or a multiple personality, she researched the subject extensively and came to the conclusion that Annie wasn't an alter ego but just another side of her developed personality, something like an imaginary friend with whom she could stockpile horrific memories, find comfort, and companionship, and store what her father referred to as her evilness.

Due to all the traumatic experiences Barb had as a child and her need to escape the pain, Annie grew stronger through the years. The two were always at odds. Every day brought another tug of war between Barb on the conservative side of an issue and Annie on the extreme liberal side. They were like oil and water, arguing over right and wrong, good and bad, fact or fiction, all or nothing. Barb had also developed Annie to protect her from the periodic physical punishment.

Barb always recognized Annie's voice in her head. Annie would speak to her as soon as her father began his pre raging episodes by criticizing, then Barb would dissociate herself or zone out, letting Annie take over and function for her. Annie couldn't stay still or hold her tongue, which always increased her father's rage. She blamed Barb's submissiveness for all the problems she had with her father, but Barb had been well trained not to resist.

In a strange way Annie was more loyal and firmly attached to her father than Barb, who thought Annie was just like him. She constantly pushed Barb toward perfection and pleasing her father so he would stop punishing them. She knew that if Barb were perfect they would gain their father's love, but there was no margin for error when it came to her father.

Barb's body slumped under the cumulative weight of her thoughts, but the seat belt stopped her from falling. She went limp for a moment when disjointed emotions from her past knifed into the center of her chest, stealing her breath and then thrusting her back into the seat. A chilling indifference spread across her ashen face. She felt like an empty shell. After a couple of seconds of reflection, Barb was able to regain some strength, check the interior of the car, and retreat deeper into her private magical space.

An image of her drawn countenance reflected from the passenger window. Barb studied her once-radiant blond locks that were now matted and greasy. She couldn't take her eyes off the weathered and empty expression on her face. The landscape raced by while she continued to examine her image, Barb contemplated all the years of physical torture, chaos, fear, and emotional beatings that had stolen her beauty, her intelligence, and most of all her spirit. To think she had once captured three beauty titles and was the homecoming queen her senior year in high school! She only judged her accomplishments as good enough when her father noticed.

Barb shook her head, forcing her painful recollections to contort and disappear back into murkiness. The gruesome images loosened their grip, but she remained on guard. Suddenly inside her mind she remembered Steven's stabbing words. He was a hyper critical and controlling man, a successful contractor by day and extremely jealous husband by night. "You would be nothing without me! Who else would put up with your ugly ass! No one would ever want you," he repeatedly told her. Those words echoed in her head, making Barb slap her hands over her ears in an attempt to suppress the noise. A single tear slid gently down Barb's cheek. Wrapped in blistering fear and anxiety, she generated a mental search for answers to why Steven had hurt her throughout their time together. No answers came. Puzzled, she reconnected to her search for what had gone wrong. Again, no answers. Annie's booming voice interrupted Barb's third attempt "Who the hell do you think you are? You know the answers; you've always known. You're hiding from them."

"Why did Steven do that?" Barb asked. Why didn't he ever accept me or need or want me?"

"You were only an object to him." Annie laughed.

Barb's head sank toward her shoulders. Shame froze her into submission. She was alert and conscious, but her body wouldn't move. She couldn't loosen Annie's emotional grip on her, nor did she want to think about her marriage any further; but Annie had other intentions. An explosion of answers shot past her denial and rained down on her.

"You weren't good enough, attractive enough for him" Annie stated. "He felt you embarrassed him in front of family and friends. You never did anything right." Annie backed off and softened her tone. "Still ignoring me?" she whispered. Barb was frozen in silence, unable to speak. "You never could keep it up," Annie said. A couple of seconds more went by with no response. "You are so stupid. Are you blind?" Annie said. "Your precious little Steven betrayed you. He isolated you from all your friends. He kept you from spending time with your family and demanded your complete allegiance. He got everything, and you got deprived. He wanted your body, not you. And to think you wouldn't go to the bathroom without his approval. Steven was just like your father. Couldn't you see it? He knew – no, he was positive you wouldn't say anything."

Annie's words tortured Barb. The puzzling stockpile of hurtful statements crumbled on top of her. *I have to stop her*, she thought, trying to encourage herself. She began to chant in her mind, *I have to stop her. I have to stop her. I must stop her at all cost.* Barb's skeletal fingers pressed harder against her temples. The pressure seemed to work, momentarily blocking the words, and her body began to relax.

Barb quickly sought to change her mental direction, but Annie refused to stop and pushed forward, describing her life between Steven and David, a lonely and confusing time. Barb went in and out of short relationships during those years. Some of them were okay, and some were outright dangerous. From fear, loneliness, and confusion she blindly walked right into another marriage hoping to erase all traces of Steven. His name was

David. An officer in the Marine Corps, David initially presented himself as the answer to all her prayers. In the beginning she had been sure that David was so different. When she first met him, he seemed perfect – attractive and charming. He was everything she ever wished for. He immediately knew her feelings, her thoughts, and her needs. He complimented and praised her, listening intently to her every word. For just a second she held those warm feelings close to help thaw out her body.

Awareness of the truth surfaced, and her mood sank like a rock in a pond. *He lied to me. He lied all those years. Oh, at first I was smitten.* Then images of David's change flashed through her mind. Bit by bit all his positive traits faded into brutality and contempt. She harbored a few nice memories of those initial days that helped her hold on during the horrifying years that followed. The truth? The truth was that her second marriage was no better than the first; they were mirror images. In a lot of ways David was slicker than Steven. Once David had gathered the information he needed on Barb, he turned her history back on her and used it to control her. She remembered how he changed right before her eyes. Fear, threats, physical punishment, rape, and deprivation became his tools for dealing with her. He was always obsessed with getting his point across. He thought it kept the relationship strong, orderly. "David's way or the highway" was his motto. "A good wife is an obedient wife." His madness increased each year, and he achieved even higher levels of control over her. His vicious behavior far surpassed Steven's in cruelty. Devoid of a heart, he never viewed Barb as anything more than a thing, an object, something to own.

Barb felt trapped in her own thinking. She tried many times to regain control of her thoughts but to no avail; her mind was controlling her. It was the voice in the left side of Barb's brain that pushed her into a deep state of self-doubt and self-judgment.

No one ever understood the massive feelings of loss and emptiness that radiated from Barb's core. When she was small and inquisitive, she never ventured into her core out of fear of what she would find. Years later, older and more wounded, she dared to go there. She searched and searched the area, finding nothing but wreckage from old emotional battles strewn everywhere. Her core, once the seat of her human qualities, was empty, scorched by battles, neglected and abandoned. Now only the ghostly faces of fear and anxiety roamed the deserted land. As a result of that venture she had pledged never to return.

Great reflections breed great questions, she thought. No one ever understood why she always had to have a man. It was the only way she knew how to get self- validation. To her, being unattached meant loneliness, nothingness. It was that nagging emptiness that propelled her into desperate relationships. "You must fill the emptiness at all costs. A women is nothing without a man," she remembered what her mother had said over and over. Barb had a driving need to find the right person to fill her inner void, yet her constant need for love and affection was never fulfilled through any of her relationships. At the beginning of each new one, she thought she had found the "right one," thought that man knew exactly what she craved. In every relationship her judgment failed and backfired. All she ever wanted was to be valued by another human being, to be loved and to be found good enough. It was not to be. She had never attained love.

Disconnecting from such distressing thoughts, she indiscriminately grabbed for anything else she could concentrate on that would allow her to numb out and lose touch with her body, but instead Barb breathed deeply, pulling herself slowly back into reality.

If David knew I was going to a treatment center, he'd fly into another one of his rages and kill me for sure this time. Barb instinctively understood that if he learned how she had betrayed him there would be nothing to stop him from punishing her severely. *There was no going back.* She physically slumped at the realization.

Barb recklessly fought to keep her hold on reality. She wanted to be conscious of sitting in the passenger seat, knowing she was safe and not back in the past. Suddenly a foreboding voice sent streams of white heat up her spine." Surprise," the foreboding voice whispered. The voice had been emanating from the left side of her brain and been present in her head since she was a young girl. The inescapable, doom-laden voice monitored her every move. It criticized her every word, contradicted her every thought, mocked every judgment and doubted every emotion. She had no authority over it. The voice directed all her feelings and behavior toward herself and her world, and any noncompliance was met with brutal consequences. She cringed from its sound.

"You better turn around! I command you. Don't dare me again! Go back before I kill you, slut," the voice threatened.

"I can't turn back," Barb's shaky voice chimed in. "My husband will hurt me, or worse, kill me. I will not let myself be held down or crippled any more, or live in fear of being murdered." Terror rose higher the more she resisted the threatening words being hurled at her. She forced her mind to escape back into her sanctuary. She no longer had any semblance of control. The voice had taken away even the least feelings of power and confidence she had. Barb was out of her league, so she cognitively retreated from yet another battle all broken and bruised. Needing to tend her wounds, she limped toward a place of protection. Maybe some safe time would help her mend. Practice told her that the deeper she withdrew into her mind, the easier it was for her to protect herself from further emotional damage.

"Let me take control for a while." Annie's voice overrode Barb's thoughts. "I can help you. I won't take that shit from him." Annie was originally produced to be wild, rebellious, and strong. She was the dark side of Barb's invalid thinking. In a crazy way Annie always took her father's side. Yet she was always there for Barb when needed.

There were other times when Annie would take over control of Barb's body and make it perform bold, independent deeds. Prevented from controlling herself, Barb cringed in fear of what was happening to her body. Annie spent most of her time in the shadows of Barb's mind, separated from the light. Annie symbolized the physical part of her that her father was after. When the body pain got too great, she stepped in to take Barb's place.

While crawling into the safety of her dark inner sanctuary to recuperate, Barb became aware that her body was functioning on its own. Viewing her body from inside her protected place, she witnessed her hand reaching for the cigarette pack on the dashboard.

"No! What are you doing? I hate smoking!" Barb yelled from deep inside her mind.

"But I love it, and you can't stop me! I'm the boss now," replied Annie, who then turned to Sandy. "Can we stop at a bar for a drink? I could really use one." Sandy reacted with surprise at the radical shift in the attitude and voice of the woman beside her. She dismissed the irrational question and returned her attention to driving the car.

Far inside her sanctuary, Barb lay nursing her wounds. She reflected on how much Annie had increased her strength and assumed greater command of her mind and body. Most of the time Annie's methods were inappropriate, but effective. Many times her behavior was downright aggressive, and with her father Annie could never hold her tongue. Barb always had a lot of explaining to do after Annie had been in control.

Barb's war-torn defenses were weakening. Her boundaries were being breached more and more frequently, and each time her pain grew. Barb had relied on Annie regularly in her childhood. She knew Annie's impulsive actions stemmed from love, but it didn't always feel like that. Annie's original mission was to contain the pain and lighten Barb's burden.

Initially Annie had not always been Barb's supporter. Barb had big trouble with her behaviors and reacted negatively toward her. Their relationship was based on conflict. Barb reflected back on all the episodes of binge drinking Annie got involved in. Annie's excessive alcoholic consumption resulted in a devastating DUI arrest two years ago. She didn't care at all, but it took all Barb's savings to pay off the lawyer. Without willful effort to retrieve any memories from that period, images flashed before her eyes. David's disapproving face appeared first. Once they were home, David's disapproval vanished into rage. He had beaten her senseless after bailing her out of jail. Barb had tried to convince him that she didn't drink and had no recollection of having done so. "It wasn't me! It wasn't me!" David beat her that whole next day and took great pleasure in refusing to believe her. He was extremely sadistic. He hurt her in many ways both physically and sexually. He killed her spirit that day. But no matter what he did to Barb, he never gained any leverage over Annie. Barb protected Annie with her silence. She could still summon up the words that David uttered while beating her. "You lying bitch." Horrible images still rich in emotion remained alive.

Interrupted by another gruesome image, she saw her father's face, and it knocked her off balance mentally. In a flash of awareness she finally connected with the fact that her two husbands were just like her father. All of them refused her any compassion or relief. Complete control of Barb was their main goal. None allowed her independent thought, feeling, or behavior that would permit her to escape physically and numb herself emotionally. She was just an object to them to be used any way they fancied. It became evident through the years that they wanted Annie not her. Annie possessed all the attributes that the three of them wanted to steal from her. Annie was wild and had passionate fire within her. If they could capture those attributes then they would fully dominate. Barb stopped comparing herself to Annie and released her mind as she took a deep breath.

Still allowing Annie to remain out front, Barb floated in a false sense of immunity within her sanctuary. She turned her attention toward a snapshot of herself as a small girl huddled in the corner of a dark closet. *I don't recall that.* Momentarily in denial she avoided its familiarity. Barb examined it further, cutting off all other distractions and straining to clear the image. *Annie. It's Annie!* For the first time in her memory she saw Annie's face. But Annie's expression worried Barb; it showed the forbidden emotion of anger.

Tearing her gaze from the picture and not wanting to deal with her latent anger, Barb opted to monitor for protection instead. She scanned the horizon of her internal asylum. Protecting self while physically recuperating was her goal at the moment. Barb stood ever on guard against any possible unknown intruders.

Fatigue began to eat at her while her defense mechanisms remained on full alert. She fully expected them to operate at their maximum level. She turned her gaze toward her outer perimeter, seeking to catch sight of her point sentry at his station. Instinct told her to stop checking and simply trust that the sentry was alert and performing his duties, but she couldn't. *Trust? Huh!* Barb's boundaries had been breached so many times that her core perimeter resembled Swiss cheese. Another trauma could occur at any point and completely devastate her. Barb never really recovered from the first terrorizing episode she had suffered as a child. Each battle disarmed or destroyed portions of her defense system. Many times her defenses had been caught off guard. She vowed never to allow that to happen again. Her ragtag army patrols every day, and she monitors all information and prepares continuously for another attack. Like a faded old photo she carries a list of all the attacks. Barb has achieved master status at hyper vigilance. She even monitors the air for any scent of danger as a wild animal would.

    Tucked safely in her private bunker, Barb found herself caught in a mental quagmire and recognized what those repeated inward journeys had cost. Annie was now in command of her mental life. Barb wondered whether she had lost the ability to regain authority over her own body and destiny. Deep down she instinctively knew that she didn't need help. She could do it alone yet without dominance and control over the rebellious Annie, she'd miss the last window of opportunity for healing. Barb wouldn't allow Annie to keep her away from another hospital. It was a given that out of loyalty to David Annie had some kind of plan to sabotage her admission. She would run back to David for more pain and punishment. Worry sunk into her consciousness, *Annie is in control.* Annie was notorious for obstructing any attempt at recovery. For her, betrayal was simply not an option.

    "I feel better now," Barb told Annie. She hesitated waiting for a reply. "Please allow me to take back control of myself. Let me back!" Barb began to plead, but Annie rebuffed her. "You weak, stupid little girl. There's not a chance in hell that you can handle what you've gotten us into!"

"Don't destroy my last chance at a normal life, you bitch!" Barb spoke in anger. Annie merely laughed. "You're as weak and worthless as they all said." Her raucous laughter grew louder in Barb's head until she felt an upsurge of unbridled wrath at her tormentor. "Stop laughing at me. I'll never let you drag me back to him. If you can't take it, then leave!" Barb caught sight of a barrage of anger emanating from Annie's arsenal. Annie and her entitled attitude were not ready to let go of power.

The unexpected mental skirmish distracted Annie's attention enough for Barb to try regaining control over her body. Gathering every ounce of willpower, she leaped at the opportunity. She caught Annie off guard, causing her to dissipate like mist in sunlight. Barb suddenly realized she'd been successful and was back in reality, though she was in the midst of a panic episode and gasping for air. *I did it!* She cheered for herself. Firmly grasping the dashboard, she held tightly to her grip on the present. Energy spent, she sat quietly, absorbing the calm that followed the successful battle with Annie.

Physically exhausted she laid her head back against the headrest and expanded her lungs to bring in a supply of oxygen to rejuvenate her brain.

Minutes later she slipped into sleep. Unknown to Barb, a dark storm front began to build deep in her mind. Relaxed, she dreamed of a brilliant blue sky, warm sunlight, and a cool breeze. It seemed just like the day of her eleventh birthday party. Overhead, billowy white clouds brought a feeling of inner peace and freedom as they traveled gently through her sleeping brain. But the approaching grayness deepened, and the wind increased. All the vital elements were uniting to form a whirlpool of twisting, colliding clouds in her mind, spitting flashes of electricity.

The storm continued its growth. Even in her sleep Barb sensed its power. With every lightning strike she saw images of people, places, and objects from her forbidden past that she was not supposed to see. The images seemed totally foreign, but the attached pain and fear felt as common as the sun in the morning. They rendered her vulnerable - powerless and defenseless. The relaxing sleep became paralyzing. Frozen as if coated with ice, she was forced to watch the parade of horrible, broken pictures from her childhood, never opened up to her before. Frustration encircled her. Morning's light was the only thing that could stop the insane process. Relief lay just on the other side of sleep, but she thought for a second that she wouldn't be able to reach it. *Wake up. Wake up right now* she commanded, as she fought for conscious control. Reality for her had always been unsafe, but now so was sleep. *No more! No more!* She screamed.

"We're not that far away," Sandy said to be reassuring. Unfortunately Barb's mind never received the message. It was too late, she had already turned her attention to analyzing the scenes that had bombarded her while she slept. There had to be an answer to her sorrow in them. She had to focus on the images and fight for consciousness at the same time. She realized that she had been the most disconnected she'd ever been from her physical self. *The key has to be here,* she thought, *but I have to wake up first.*

Barb awoke, frightened at the sound of her heart pounding in her ears. Disoriented and startled, she grabbed her face to verify that she still was in control of her body. She found herself huddled against the cold car door, held upright only by her seat belt. She made the effort to regain her composure before she turned to look at Sandy, whose tenderly warm and supportive hand was pressing against her shoulder.

Since she first began entertaining thoughts of treatment again, Barb had been steadily separating more often from her body and losing more time. Treatment always brought on depression, fear, anxiety, and cruel reflections of past pain. Other people were increasingly aware of her unrelenting depression, and asked too many questions. She was unable to hide the devastating effect of the surfacing symptoms of past abuse. She had grown so tired of fighting, both inside and outside herself that she finally accepted the idea of being broken – defective and damaged beyond repair. She was drowning in misery and too tired to engage in the ritual dance with her symptoms. She had to do something. She decided to give in, reach out for help and work the treatment no matter the cost. Every nerve in her body throbbed as they traveled ever closer to the hospital.

A cutting voice derailed Barb's train of thought as Annie interrupted. "You know once those charlatans find out you're crazy, they'll lock you up and throw away the key! You'll never get out!" Fear climbed up Barb's spine like a scared cat scaling a tree. She quickly wiped away the waxy sweat that beaded her upper lip, hoping that Sandy wouldn't see she was reacting to an internal voice.

"You can't do this! Don't be a fool!" Annie said. "It isn't normal to have a voice talking in your head. They won't understand and won't listen. They'll hurt you just the way the others did. Bitch, get her to stop this car now!" Annie warned. Barb attempted to quell her meddling racket by clenching her teeth, but Annie's voice slipped through. "If you follow through with this stupid idea, he'll hurt you again. This time David will kill you for sure, just the way your father almost did." For the first time Barb saw that Annie was holding out on her just as she had kept secrets from her throughout childhood. For a second Barb recoiled in fear before pushing her shoulders back and raising her head. "Tell me what you know Annie, tell me right now!" She crossed her arms over her chest and embraced the silence while waiting for an answer, but none came. Five minutes passed, and her anxiety nearly doubled. She started to cringe as though she had done something wrong.

"I beg of you!" Barb appealed, using a different approach with a softer tone. Her anxiety increased when there was still no answer. Her pulse quickened as she frantically searched her mental files for bits and pieces of childhood scenes. She had to discover all the buried memories so Annie couldn't blackmail her with them. *Maybe I missed something.* The frenzied search produced nothing useable. Pain pierced the right side of her face as the vision of a heavy oak closet door opening crashed into her consciousness. She had a physical sensation of being dragged toward it. The weight of the images sat heavily upon her chest, and all the air escaped from her lungs. "Here's your answer," taunted Annie. Barb had the sensation of a large hand pressing on her private parts. Gasping, Barb tried to regroup. She set her feet against the floorboard of the car and forced air back into her lungs. *No, that cannot be him, he wouldn't.* Tears formed in her eyes. She took a moment and just sat, paralyzed, recharging her batteries.

With her external vision monitoring reality while she dealt with Annie, Barb caught a glimpse of a roadside blue hospital sign. It read fifteen miles. She had little time left to decode the mental visions. She turned her focus back inside her head. That wasn't real. I made it up, she told herself, increasing her denial. The pain continued to expand. Annie reached out from within the darkest cavern of Barb's mind and confirmed her worst fears. "Yes, your own father. He did it and did it often" Annie said.

"You didn't make it up. That's a bad joke. It all happened, and you left me there. You ran away. I loved you, Barb, and you abandoned me. I took it all" Annie stated. "You left me with Daddy and let him hurt me. He hurt me bad. The next day you acted as if it never happened." Even worse, you denied my existence. You just plain rejected me." Barb's chin dropped to her chest from the shock of what she was hearing. *Had I hated myself that much? Did I disown myself?*

The car slowed and turned into the long driveway. It traveled to the entrance in the back of the large, two-story building. A sign read: Admissions.

"Barb, we're here!" Sandy, her longtime friend who'd been driving, uttered with a sense of achievement.

What was left of Barb just sat there motionless and unresponsive.

Chapter 2

Pain

With Annie's words still ringing in her ears, Barb sat still as the noise of the engine stopped. Sandy patted her arm. "You wait here, and I'll make sure this is the right place," she said.

Barb watched her friend walk up the flower bordered sidewalk and disappear through a nondescript entrance. Anxious and scared, she remained obediently in the car for what seemed hours but in reality was only minutes. *Maybe it's not such a good idea. Maybe I'm overreacting. Maybe I made a horrible decision,* doubt invaded her thoughts. *Did I make the right decision? Should I run?* She turned toward the driver's side, and her eyes locked on the ignition. *Shit, no keys.* She frantically searched for another means of escape.

Barb shifted in her seat so she could see through the big glass entrance door. Safety was always a dominant concern. *Will I be safe?*

"You don't have to do this." Annie spoke in an unusually soft and supportive manner and broke in on her thoughts. "Great, another country heard from. So you've returned." Barb jabbed at her.

"Don't kid around. This is serious," Annie begged. "You're about to be locked up again. Have you forgotten the pain at the last hospital?" she asked.

At the mention of hospitals the veil of denial began to lift from Barb's mind. This wasn't her first hospitalization, but she had been blocking those unpleasant memories.

Barb was the good little girl who always protected the family name. That loyalty cost her more than it ever did the others. Instead of having found safety or protection at the hospitals, she encountered disbelief, disillusionment, and more trauma and misunderstanding. *No one ever understood.* With each admission Barb experienced an increase in the intensity of her internal upheaval and had less ability to hide her symptoms from the outside world. A surge of angry feelings surfaced, leading her to confront Annie.

"Many of my past visits to the funny farm are your fault, if you remember correctly."

Waves of bright images of her other admissions began to dance across Barb's mental screen. She gathered her thoughts. On the eve of this new admission, she had many more bits of childhood memories and adult traumas than she'd had during her last hospitalizations. "It was you who wouldn't stop drinking."

"Do you blame me?" Annie retorted.

"Shut up and let me talk," Barb said. Then she grimaced as she reviewed the severity of past experiences in hospitals from storage areas deep within the caverns of her mind. "It was you who attacked that storekeeper. It was you who always stole things. It was you who picked up all those men and acted out for your own gratification. It was you who always pissed off David." She also recalled graphic accounts of all the acting-out behaviors Annie used to cut off Barb's pain. "It was me, so what," Annie admitted.

Barb's concept of time collapsed under the weight of endless scary images. The all too familiar picture show seemed to have no beginning, no end, and no boundaries. These haunting images had invaded every aspect of her life and reduced her ability to function. The frequency of such episodes had increased twofold every year since her thirtieth birthday. She never told anyone her true perceptions or the secrets she held about her abuse, her life, or herself. Barb marveled for a second at how she'd taken care of a home, a child, and a job while hiding her pain from everyone.

Keeping pain at bay became all-consuming. The effort to control the repetitive, intrusive episodes for so many years drained off every last drop of her energy and strength. Things eventually reached a point where she was unable to carry out any of her responsibilities. She could no longer pretend, pain had finally won.

Denial came to the rescue. Barb's right hand unconsciously scratched at the dry skin on her left elbow, the movement allowed her to protect her chest against possible attack. She felt empty and worthless. *I guess I got the type of life I deserved.* Head bowed in defeat, her lonely figure remained motionless in the car. She was jerked back to consciousness by the opening of the car door.

"It's okay; you can come in now. This is the right place," Sandy said. Barb took a deep breath and climbed out. Hyper vigilance flaring, she continued to find her surroundings suspect, her walk slowed and labored. A smiling stranger held the door as she stepped through the hospital's entrance. She froze in mid step as she registered the agonizing sound of the door's bolt sliding noisily into the steel frame that surrounded it.

It's done Barb sighed, remembering the words her father had yelled at her throughout her life: "You're crazy." Now the clicking bolt confirmed her worse fears; she was truly crazy.

Barb quickly scanned the cold, lifeless sitting room that lay in front of her. Her senses were functioning at an acute protection level. She found the air musty and the light too brilliant. The furniture was worn by the hundreds of human bodies that had sat there, and a yellow film of age dimmed the brightness of the white walls. The floor was highly polished to hide the phantom path created by all the hurting souls who paraded past the admission desk. She breathed in the sterile smell covering the stench of fear.

"If you would take a seat, I'll be with you as fast as possible." Barb took a step back as the unnoticed figure from behind the admission desk addressed her. Unable to respond, she moved swiftly to the dilapidated couch set against the far wall. It would give her the best vantage point from which to monitor the room. She scanned the area to reassure herself that she was safe. Barb sat there, expressionless, and frozen, determined to contain the emotional upheaval rising inside her. Her mind reviewed the events that had occurred during her trip to the hospital. She couldn't remember a time in her life when she'd experienced such a concentrated assault by recollections. Something deep inside didn't want her to be admitted. As fear increased she began to twist into the position of a child waiting to be punished. The chill of isolation wrapped itself around her like a familiar blanket. Sitting alone for an extended period stretched her patience thin. The admission process was an impersonal and time-consuming task. Feelings of being trapped filled Barb's mind. She rejected such thoughts, knowing they would make her uncomfortable.

Barb had been walking a fine line between sanity and insanity for many years. Being a wife made her feel like an acrobat performing on a high wire. One slip, one incorrect move, and it might be her last. Her second husband allowed no room for imperfection. Day after day it grew harder to keep her balance. Constantly anticipating failure, she'd given up on achieving success or pleasing David. He was never satisfied. Barb glanced at the emergency exit door numerous times, a need to escape stirring within her. "Go ahead, do it! Run! They couldn't catch you!" Annie shouted at her. Barb's muscles tightened, preparing her body to flee. Was this her time for recovery? Maybe she'd misjudged herself. Could she fight the pain this time or respond as she had in the other programs and continue to hide her secrets. She wondered how she'd tolerate the therapist's constant observation and invasion of her inner world. Would the program help her violent pain or make her withdraw as all the others had? Could anyone stop her need to isolate herself? She shook her head vigorously to interrupt the flow of those thoughts. The self-questioning had to end before it turned into a full-blown emotional blaming cycle. Barb spoke to herself with a sense of urgency. *I will survive. My phony life of lies has to stop now.*

Barb continued to sit motionless like a stone gargoyle on a building. Locked in time, her mind reflected warmly on her only true friend. Once her worst enemy, Annie had been transformed into a companion, a valuable confederate - an ally who was always there for her, especially when her father locked her in the closet. She had created Annie in her mind to be ever present, ever consistent. But somehow Annie grew in strength as her father's abuse increased. She was the only marker Barb had to let her know she was surviving the torture she endured. Annie performed many services. She held all the pain and negative emotions Barb was unable to integrate. She helped her deny what had been happening during her childhood.

Annie was that aspect of herself that helped keep her equilibrium. Without her, Barb's ability to adapt and function would have been impossible. At times her father and husbands had used Annie against her, yet it was Annie who pulled her through the most violent episodes. Barb counted on her to be a shield to ward off pain.

Barb giggled to herself at the idea of creating Annie. She used her skillfully, but thinking of her now helped Barb confirm the paradox she found herself in. Barb had traveled all this distance for a chance at recovery and freedom. The program was an opportunity to stop being controlled by her intrusive posttraumatic symptoms. She was coming to the hospital to embrace a new method that might mean a fresh beginning, another start, and a chance for health. That she might lose Annie in the process brought on a flash of fear, but if her efforts were successful, they wouldn't walk out of the program together.

Barb closed her eyes, trying to separate herself from reality and a wave of negativism. The possibility of escape raged in her mind. *Run* streamed across her mental screen. She slapped the left side of her head and countered with, *Stop reacting in fear. You're here to get better.* Then self-doubts set in again. *Why am I so inconsiderate, so selfish, only thinking of me? How can I just let Annie go when she has been such a loyal companion? Do I really want to exist without the only person I know? How much longer can I last like this?* Doubts bounced of her mental walls, and fighting them let confusion invade Barb's mind. All possible answers seemed to be blocked. Suddenly hyper vigilance rose from the flames of that confusion, and Barb's primitive need to escape grew stronger. Her eyes darted back and forth behind half-closed lids while her body cringed.

Feeling physically confined as an onslaught of images flashed by, Barb recalled the first time she neutralized pain without Annie. It started with an innocent dare from a blind date at a fraternity party. That night, drinking was her attempt to fit in socially, but Barb had not been ready for the numbing effect alcohol had on her pain. She didn't need Annie. Her first solo feeling of independence was fake, a chemical reaction. But as Barb advanced in age, Annie's strength advanced also. After that Annie stepped in and adopted alcohol as her own throughout Barb's college years. The more Barb drank, the less effect it had on her companion, so she raised the stakes by combining alcohol with various drugs to bring back her original experience of freedom. To her peers she seemed to consume any available chemical in the name of socializing. Inwardly Barb was on a mission to separate herself from Annie, yet Annie seemed to navigate around the chemical walls of numbness and take over. Annie became the life of the party crowd, while Barb continued to seek newer and newer combinations of drugs. What she thought would be a chemical savior turned out to provide only a false front. It seemed that times free of her companion grew shorter and shorter. In those days Barb worked hard to escape her. In spite of all her efforts, the next morning Annie was there when she awoke. Barb could escape situations and people in her mind but never Annie.

All through college and until she was twenty-eight, the tug of war between them developed into a no-win situation. No matter how far Barb attempted to run, how inappropriate her behaviors were, or how many chemicals she ingested Annie remained ever-present. What Barb finally understood was that in uniting with Annie, she was able to achieve a higher level of numbness when facing the violent punishment inflicted by her husbands. The penalty for her numb-seeking behavior was addiction to alcohol, drugs, and risky behavior patterns that got out of control. As sick as it may sound, Barb remembered enjoying the effects of multiple addictions. Now, sitting in the admission area, she finally understood that the dangerous game she played with her pain had to stop, or she would die. Barb's vigilant third eye warned her of an approaching figure clad in white. She didn't even raise her head to look, but her hands turned cold and wet.

"Would you like to come with me?" the nurse said. I'll start your admission. Barb rose and followed her without question, staring at the back of the nurse's white shoes. She was escorted into a small room and asked to sit in front of a desk. She was uneasy with the closeness of the walls. Her heart rate accelerated. In the room's dim light the uniformed figure of the nurse reminded her of the reason she'd made the long trek to the hospital.

"So why are you here?" The nurse asked beginning the assessment interview. Barb's posture became as erect as if she were a prisoner defending herself against an accusing interrogator. She had just spent the five hours of the trip reviewing her past, and here she was being asked to face it all over again. Barb took care to answer the nurse's questions in very general and evasive terms.

Annie whispered within Barb's head, "Don't tell her anything. She doesn't care what you think. She'll only believe you're crazy. You're a fool. Sudden insanity has made you forget what will happen if you go through with this."

"What are you, blind?" Barb answered. "I'm already dead. This is my final chance. If it doesn't work out we'll both be dead. I can't live this way anymore." She turned her attention back to the admission nurse and hoped for some validation. She searched the woman's face, looking for a modicum of understanding of her internal battle and saw no negative responses there.

As the interrogation continued, the nurse's questions centered on Barb's childhood. Searching her memories made her jumpy. She felt as if the walls were moving in on her. All of a sudden the idea of safety leaped into her consciousness. *Will they protect me or not? Do I take a chance?* A rapid, chaotic hunt started in her brain for an answer to the question of how not to get disappointed or hurt again. The pace of her thoughts began to accelerate. Her mind intercepted an urgent message from her body to run.

"Get away before the nurse realizes you're nuts and locks us up for good," Annie whispered. Barb grew extremely annoyed at her attempt to take control. It wasn't the time to get into an internal argument with her. The nurse was only four feet away and looking right into her eyes. Barb's head was pounding. Her level of fear increased as she fought off the desire to take refuge in her sacred internal territory and withdraw from reality. Her right leg started bouncing up and down involuntarily. She leaned her arm hard on her right thigh to cover up its jerky movement.

"How was your relationship with your father while you were growing up?" asked the nurse. A large knot formed in Barb's throat. She hesitated and then spoke reluctantly as she broke eye contact. "My father loved me! I was the apple of his eye. He took me everywhere with him. It was always just the two of us." Tears welled up in her eyes, but Barb kept her face void of expression. Detached from her true emotions, she continued to answer, verbally painting a picture of her father as a loving yet troubled man who was secretive, controlling, and lonely. To ward off the hurt of her troubled relationship with him, Barb focused on determining whether the nurse had caught the incongruence of her answers. As she gazed at the wall, she experienced the sensation of a large, invisible finger pressing on her lips. A low sound filled her head and she disconnected from reality.

Her father's voice traveled through her thoughts like a gust of wind. *Shhh, don't tell. They're trying to break us up. I loved you.* Barb's mind froze; she uttered no response. Again her father's voice sounded a warning. *You know what will happen if you tell.*

Barb recognized the terrorizing threat that had just surfaced in her consciousness, paralyzing her vocal cords. She was drowning in a pool of fear. While her mind scrambled for damage control, the blood rushed from her head. Barb dared not adjust her position, thinking any movement would call attention to her internal conflict and her need to avoid betraying her father. Her eyes locked on her hands that were now gripping both thighs. She begged herself, *Hang in there; hang in there; don't leave. Oh God, please let me stay.* The nurse's voice cut through her mental chaos.

"And your mother – how was your relationship with her? As fast as fear had entered, it withdrew, replaced by an upsurge of bitter anger. Barb's defenses banded together to form her answer.

"All my life it was very strained. I could never understand her behavior toward me. We didn't get along, not at all. She was critical of everything I did or said. It seemed as though I couldn't do anything right. She made me feel we were in competition, yet against my better judgment I always took care of her when she was in need. I didn't deserve to be treated that way." Barb hesitated, took a slow, deep breath and continued. "She was supposed to protect me, not reject me."

"What was she supposed to protect you from?" The nurse's ears pricked up.

"I'm sorry I said that," Barb answered.

"That's okay, just go on," the nurse reassured her.

"Well, she was never a mother to me. I really think she hated me. We haven't talked since I left that house at age eighteen. I was a disappointment to her."

"My parents were forever arguing." she reported now more controlled. "Sometimes my father hit my mother. She told me she'd made him mad or done something wrong and deserved the beating." Barb's bottled-up anger intensified, but she continued making excuses in an effort to offset her previous statements. "She always defended him, and I felt very sorry for her. I guess that's why she drank so much. My father needed to feel superior and in control at all times. He was always so serious. I think it was his work that made him angry. He never tolerated anything but perfection, and I never measured up to his unreasonable standards." Barb all of a sudden heard her own words and knew she was minimizing the extent of her parent's dysfunction.

Another message escaped to the surface of her mind. "Run, run, run! He's furious," echoed Annie's voice.

"You have gone too far!" Her father's magnified voice interrupted. Barb's jaw muscle tightened as she felt a sharp pain at the back of her neck. She connected with Annie by forcing her ragged nails into the palms of her hands. Her body stiffened. Entangled in the internal clash, she heard the sound of the nurse's voice seem to fade. She fought to stay in the here and now, but she was trapped between a frightening pseudoreality and an enticing invitation to run. She was being torn apart by powerful opposing forces and had to make a choice between two worlds. For many years Barb had been devoted to an inner world that represented loneliness, isolation, and darkness. The outer world represented life and hope but always meant pain. Never being allowed to make her own decisions had come back to haunt her. The more she tried to decide, the more confusion flared.

"Damn it, let me handle it. You're going to get us killed." A recognizable plea from Annie broke through the dense smoke of emotional ferment.

Though Annie had saved her many times, giving her control in this situation was not a good idea. She hoped with all her might that someone else would intervene and make the decision for her. Throughout her life other people instructed her how to think, act, and feel. Now every decision meant a battle within. Each choice held its own attractive seductiveness. For an instant she gave serious consideration to submitting to Annie's offer. Barb straightened, lifted her head, and mentally recanted the proposal. *No way! No way in hell! This time I have to do it on my own.*

"Are you all right? Is there something I can do for you?" the nurse asked. The warmth of a concerned hand on her arm forced her back to reality.

"No, I...I was just thinking about your last question" she said, quickly regaining her composure.

The nurse continued questioning Barb on many areas of concern: use of alcohol or drugs, problems sleeping, fluctuations in her weight, eating habits, mood swings, flashbacks, and nightmares. Barb didn't remember what she answered because her mind was embroiled in conflict. She continued to have difficulty concentrating on the questions. Part of her mental energy focused on the conversation, and the other part concentrated on the chaos in her brain. Still sickened by the threats and battling with Annie for control, she found her ability to speak coherently diminished. Her lips were dry and bloodless. Barb hadn't experienced such a difficult episode in years. Her body quivered to its core as the unresolved pain from the past reached her threshold of endurance.

"You've really done it now. He'll rain down his fury on us. Stop! Don't say another word, bitch," Annie screamed in an attempt to persuade her. Barb rejected the statement and lashed out at the nurse.

"Are we done with this?" Patience abandoned her. She just wanted either to leave or be admitted to the program.

I think we've finished the admission interview. I just have to get your paperwork together. Please, Mrs. Freeman, return to the waiting area, and I'll come and get you," the nurse said, hoping to reduce her new patient's frustration.

Barb remained on guard while she waited; doubt again crawled into her mind. *Is what I said real, or did I make it up?* She had been living a lie so long that it had become reality. Repeated negative messages were so constant that she eventually adopted them as her own, though they originated from an evil source – her father. After years of hearing ugly messages, she broke down and accepted them. They became her beliefs and values. A monster existed deep inside her that periodically emerged unchecked. She was defenseless against it.

Suddenly Barb realized she wasn't alone. Her senses carefully examined the waiting room. Her peripheral vision caught sight of a hideous shadow moving across the wall to her left. She turned quickly to confront it, but there was nothing there. Her ears searched for reassuring sounds from the nurse that would allow her some sense of safety. But when Barb heard her down at the end of the hallway, her heartbeat got louder, and her attentiveness became hyper vigilance. She was petrified. At that point she understood she had awakened the evil force from its lair. It was starved for revenge. The monster whose job it was to track betrayal was moving in on its prey, and she was the prey. Barb had opened too many secrets. Her behavior would not be tolerated.

Barb waited patiently, though the minutes slowed to a crawl. She remained alone in the waiting room, feeling as exposed as a hunk of raw meat suspended from a limb of an oak tree. The shadows of doubt increased in her mind, and she allowed them to grow into self-questioning. *Have I made a grave mistake and betrayed all of them? Or slipped during the interview?* She knew the monster within heard everything she said to the nurse. An aroma of death penetrated the open receptors of her olfactory system. She had to remain alert, knowing that if she rested even for a second, the consequences might be worse than ever. Barb honestly answered her question with another: *If I have to live like this for the rest of my years, then I don't want to live.* Without warning she was jerked back into reality by the nurse, who said, "I can take you to the program now."

    Startled, Barb stroked her face to verify that she was still awake and alive. Stiff from remaining in her protective position, she slowly stood, picked up her musty old suitcases, and followed the woman in white. As they left the waiting room she glanced back at the glass door to the outside for the last time. She took a deep breath and passed through another locked door.

Chapter 3

Discovery

    Barb's anxiety increased with each step as she moved blindly down the long hospital corridor behind the ghost-like figure of the nurse. Retreat and escape were no longer options. The unfamiliarity of the hospital held her in a dream-like state. Time had lost its importance, and her senses were at the height of alertness. She directed all her energy reserves into the system whose mission was to scan for danger through monitoring her surroundings. Cold fear draped itself over her. At the moment she yearned for the warmth and protection of one of her grandmother's handmade wool shawls. She'd felt safe when she had been with her grandmother. She was the only one who ever understood her. Before moving on Barb bowed her head for a second to honor the memory of her dead grandmother. A flood of shame at her present act of betrayal rushed through her and pushed away the enveloping fear.

    "Let me take over," came Annie's whisper, hinting at escape. "I'll help you out of this mess. I can handle these people. Don't you know you're breaking all the rules? They said they would kill us. Please give me control."

    "Can't you see that I'm busy"? Barb snapped back. She was keeping a reasonable distance behind the nurse. The space reassured her that Annie couldn't be overheard.

    Electrical pulses rushing through Barb's entire being started her eyelids flickering at a rapid rate as she entered the buried archives of her mind. Because of the sensitivity of the material, everything she now viewed appeared to be happening in slow motion. The nurse in front of her moved like a character in an old-time movie. She remembered her father taking her to one when she was very young.

All of a sudden Barb froze in her tracks like a deer catching the scent of danger. Frightening waves of overwhelming emotions smothered her. Out of the corner of her inner eye she caught a distorted glimpse of the backs of aged theater seats and smelled an odor of mildewed upholstery. Her mind burned with more fragments of alarming images. *Oh, my God. Not more. Not now. I cannot tolerate another flashback. It's the smell.* Barb cupped her hand over her nose to block it. Yet a grotesque impression of being soiled crept across her skin. She stiffened defensively as if to repel an attack and fought to regain a link with reality. *He loved me. I was his favorite. I was special to him. He told me so,* she thought, hoping that confirming her father's lies would halt the onslaught of painful scenes.

"You don't have to go through this. Come home! Let me get you out of this fix. You've never been able to handle this kind of situation. I've always done your dirty work. Please," Annie begged.

The nurse stopped and turned to face her. For a second Barb thought she had heard Annie's voice.

"Is something wrong?"

"My leg got a cramp," Barb was quick to answer.

"You need to keep up. We're almost there, and then you can rest.

Rest, how funny is that?

Barb realized that the badge she was about to receive for her long walk was the honor of facing her own secrets. It was now or never. Her expectations had grown enormously ever since she phoned the hospital to verify admission. Somehow, deep inside she had developed expectations that the treatment program had magical powers, and help was just down the hallway.

Confusion clogged her mental pathways as she attempted to search for a way out of this situation. *If this doesn't work, I'm dead. I'm dead anyway if David finds out I'm in treatment again.* Barb kept pace behind the nurse, sort of using her as a shield to protect her from unexpected attack. Catching her off balance was always his way. She could remember David laughing when he was done with her, saying "I do it for shock value. It keeps you on your toes." A list of all the threats David threw at her flashed through her mind. Simultaneously, a second-level alert rang in her head.

Her father's voice sought to change her decision to get help and undermine her hope. "It's not too late to save yourself. This place is just like all the others. You can't trust them. They only make you worse. There's danger here. Be a good girl and go home! You're my little princess, and she wouldn't betray me! Run, run for your life!"

Barb sank under an avalanche of shame, yet she defiantly continued to forge ahead on her trek of betrayal. Using all her powers, Barb just ignored the presence of the voice. Every bit of her strength went into completing each footstep, though every inch of her progress broke another piece of her heart.

Attempting to gain control of her thoughts, Barb concentrated on details of the program. She had heard so much about this treatment center's specialized mode of stabilization. Previous programs had dealt only with her symptoms. *Yeah, those places were just Band-Aid therapy. Do it and come back again in two months.* They did nothing to abate the emptiness and pain that was rampant within her. No program had penetrated the depths of her endless darkness. Previous therapists retreated when touching the fringes of her limitless pit of hurting. The other programs unintentionally separated her from her only avenues for numbing her symptoms and replaced them with nothing. Without her tools she became vulnerable; her pain grew, and she was triggered into relapse. *"Just don't use today." Ha! Great philosophy, but it doesn't work when I happen to be the one who's being used. The therapists took away my addictions and left me exposed to all the things causing my agony.* She paused and then continued thinking. *No matter how many times I tried to explain, they just couldn't see.* Barb cried quietly, but her tears went unnoticed. The other programs couldn't or wouldn't work with her truth. Therapists said "You're in denial and defocusing from your addiction; you need to get sober, save the trauma work for later with your outpatient therapist."

But later never came. Barb's outpatient therapist knew even less how to deal with her underlying trauma issues than the dual diagnosis program she had just left. The only way Barb could convey her anguish was to act out. Acting out was also her attempt at inhibiting effects of the medications they gave her. She remembered most of her past inpatient experiences through a drug-induced fog. *No one had understood what I was going through. No staff even cared.* She had used all that money and time in hospital programs that didn't understand she had spent her life fighting to survive, to live rather than fighting to recover.

The further she walked, the more hyper vigilant of her environment she became. The hallway seemed to grow in size as though she were seeing it through a child's eyes. Then Annie intruded, "Bitch. You better listen to me! Let me help you. You're thinking crazy." Barb answered her with silence. "You're pissing me off," Annie said. "Don't you know what your actions will cost us? Death, stupid! Stop right now! You've never done anything right when it comes to these places. Let me in; give me control now!" Barb flinched but kept moving on. The nurse turned, extended her hand toward Barb, palm up. "Wait here," she said, and then quickly disappeared around the corner.

Barb felt abandoned and ached with loneliness. Small phantomlike flames of fear flared up from deep within her, urging her to flee, run, escape. But her legs turned to cement, dead weight. Terrified and down to her last options, she reached out to her old companion and whispered, "Annie, okay, I was wrong. Please."

"What do you want? Can't you see I am busy?" Annie replied in a cocky tone.

"Help me."

Annie came back with, "Help you? What for? After what you have done to me and how you've used me? Do I look stupid all of a sudden?"

"Help me stay here," Barb begged. Only silence filled the space in her skull while tension ran through her veins.

"Help me stay here, we deserve a chance," she begged again.

Time stood still, but there was no answer.

"You want me to do what?" Annie said, taken off balance by the receipt of her first true validation from Barb.

Barb pleaded her case:

Hell, if you don't help me, we're both dead, David or not. So if you won't help me, if you won't be my ally, then you will be considered my enemy like all the rest. Understand with that stance, you'll be my first target once I get into treatment. I won't let you wreck it for me. History and familiarity will not save you. It is your decision.

The admissions nurse appeared from around the corner and motioned for Barb to follow.

Barb smiled outwardly to disguise her emotional conflict and the ensuing damage. She did not want to be discovered. The pressure grew. She lifted her head in triumph as she glimpsed the twin metal doors of the unit. Painted above them was the phrase: "The path to recovery is through emotions." She recognized it from the literature they'd sent. She thought she was at the end of her long, agonizing journey, but in fact it was only the beginning. The mere thought of captivity sent waves of electricity up her spine. Control had always been a major issue, and this was a critical point in her life. She was about to give up control to the program. Her posture slumped as she momentarily doubted her decision.

Snapping back to reality, she caught sight of a program nurse talking to the admissions nurse while looking over her shoulder at Barb. The "look" from the nurse made Barb feel transparent as though she could look right through her, feeling as if she were on display made her posture remain rigid. Sensing Barb's fear the program nurse moved toward her and pressed her hand gently against Barb's bony arm.

"You're safe now. No one will hurt you. Come in. We understand the fear you must be experiencing. It's okay; we can help."

"Empty promises," Annie interrupted. "If you believe that, you're a bigger fool than they said."

Barb stopped short of stepping through the cold steel doors leading into the program area. The look on her face was like that of one about to be eaten by an ogre. She tried to move her legs, but they didn't seem to register the message. The admitting nurse approached Barb after dropping off her papers at the desk. She perceived Barb's hesitation and discomfort. She walked over to Barb and gently took her hand and led her through the doors.

Letting go of her, the nurse attempted to comfort by saying, "You'll be safe now. Remember, it already happened; it is not happening. It won't happen here. You'll be protected now." A pause ensued as the nurse peered into her eyes looking for validation. "I have to leave you and go back to my station. You are in good hands, she reassured. Barb watched as she faded out of sight down the hallway. The doors closed.

A voice invaded her few seconds of quiet. "Wow! Are you buying this? Wake up! It is all bullshit? She's lying to you. Can't you see that?" Annie warned.

Tears of pain filled Barb's eyes as the internal conflict ripped her into smaller pieces, but she wasn't leaving. She was here to stay. On the other hand Annie, the opposite side of her mind, wanted out, wanted to escape the flood of old emotions immediately because being at the program was a pure act of betrayal punishable by execution. Though Barb felt like retreating into the furthest point inside her mind and never returning, she hung on, determined to give the program a chance. Preceded by an ominous stillness, the second level of alert sounded.

"Go no further! I'll kill you if you tell our secret. I'll always be present to hear everything you say. There's no escaping me!" Her father's authoritarian voice erupted in her brain.

Jolted, Barb began to slip away mentally. She struggled to remain in contact with reality and fought by resorting to her usual behavior patterns in response to his threats. Trapped in betrayal and guilt, her first reaction was to curl up in a corner of the room. She resisted the temptation and went to sit in a chair by the window. If she acted out as usual, the program would have her number. She had to keep focused.

"Don't you freeze on me!" Annie commanded. "You'll get sucked into a memory. Get up and move!" She'd understood Barb's weakness since childhood.

Holding still any longer would make her vulnerable to a flashback, and reliving the past could unmask her to the program staff. Someone at the desk or nursing station might recognize her "I'm fine" ploy. She got up and walked around, appearing to be orienting herself to the area. Meanwhile the silent battle raged between reacting to her internal reality and not being discovered by the external world. *That seems to be the theme of my life, so what's new?* "Just keep walking," she muttered. Barb's entire frame shook in fear with each stride. Her gut ached, and her head felt light. She kept walking. Flashing images drifted through her consciousness. She kept walking. Shame weighed heavily in her muscles. She ignored the weight and kept walking.

In midstride her pale green eyes locked in on a shiny doorknob. It could be the focal point that would help her numb out the pain and fear surging in her body. But immediately she was interrupted by the nurse's sudden question.

"Where did you go?" She asked.

"Just thinking," Barb said. "You have to go away to think, don't you?"

"You think an awful lot," the nurse remarked. "Well, it's time for me to go. My shift is over, but I'm leaving you in safe hands for the night." "I'll be back in the morning." She turned and then looked back again stating "Try not to go too far, in your thinking that is." Her statement puzzled Barb at first and made her think she had been discovered already. But she got the pun and let out a quick forced laugh.

The double doors opened for the nurse and they slowly closed after her. The narrowing space between them beckoned Barb to slip through and dash for freedom. Gazing at the doors, Barb heard the sound of the tumbler clicking shut. It was a done deal. *Trapped again.*

"You've done it now!" A pissed-off Annie proclaimed. "I won't help you anymore. You're on your own." Suddenly the interior of Barb's head went black. A stillness, a silence she had never before experienced asserted itself. She was lost in a sense of emptiness, once again rejected and abandoned for trying to help herself. She didn't know what she'd do without Annie. She was firmly committed to following through on her decision to seek recovery no matter what the cost, even if it cost her Annie.

"Ha! She's gone." The sound of her father's voice sliced through the left side of her brain. "You're mine. You can't fight me now. Remember what I'm capable of."

A flashback of her father slamming her against a wall replayed in her mind. Barb panicked. Her mind, body, and spirit had separated, Her thinking and emotions were in full defensive mode. Her worlds were completely divided now.

A staff member was ready to orient Barb to program policies and procedures. She mechanically went through what Barb viewed as the "admission dance," then escorted her to her assigned room. Following the technician, she became painfully aware of the other women in the program staring at her as she made her way across the main floor, down a hallway, past group rooms, and finally arrived at her sleeping quarters.

Still behind the tech, Barb stopped short of the doorway and lowered her head, resisting the impulse to look in either direction thus avoiding the gawking eyes of the other women. There is no way she could take their visual assessment right now. Other people's opinions always played a major role in how she thought, acted, or felt. But she wanted to operate on her own and keep her word to herself about treatment. She'd already been judged too much. The judgments she carried around were bad enough. No more were needed.

The tech finished unlocking the door and went in, disappearing into the darkened room as though swallowed. Taking a deep breath, Barb raised her head, crossed the threshold, and entered right behind her. The hall light flooded into the bedroom, overtaking the darkness, but it barely illuminated the room's furnishings. Squinting, Barb rapidly took a mental inventory. There were two wooden-framed beds with eight-inch institutional green mattresses on top, two small imitation wood desks, one big closet, and a half-opened door that led to the small but adequate bathroom, where her nose registered a strong smell of chlorine. She'd had bathroom issues her whole life and never could figure out why. *It must have been an issue in my childhood.* To increase her feeling of safety Barb selected the left bed which was farthest from the windows. There she would have good line of sight around the room. Positioning was so critical when out of your own environment. She had now designated her space, a small amount of ownership.

As soon as the tech left, Barb became task-driven to forestall thinking of the mess she had caused. She made her bed. While working she was overcome by a sense of being alone and helpless. *Is this room a self-inflicted prison cell? How cold and sterile it is.* Shaking off such negative thoughts, she went back to putting her stuff away. She then pulled her hand-quilted bedcover and matching pillow from the bottom of her suitcase and place them on her bed. Barb stood back casting a critical eye at her work. *Now it is my bed.*

It was late by the time she completed settling in. Barb closed her door and turned off the lights. She didn't even change her clothes but simply flopped onto the bed and pulled the bedspread over her body. She curled up under it to give herself a sense of being protected. Finally gaining some assurance of safety, she allowed her eyes to close.

Relaxing for a second, Barb was transported back to the years when she was a high-school cheerleader. Memories that had been buried deep within came alive again. Even in the dark a smile of self-satisfaction came across her face, which was not a customary expression for her. It was a short-lived period of her life, but she cherished it as her best years. It was a time when other people looked up to her. She remembered walking through the hallways at high school not worrying if people were looking at her. People even spoke to her spontaneously. Her peers regarded her as successful, and she presented herself to her schoolmates as dedicated, proud, sociable, and smart. In those days she was a person who had demonstrated confidence in herself and walked with her head up. Barb was never allowed to be that way at home. Her father would have killed her had he seen that kind of blatantly independent behavior. But in order for her to accomplish her goals, she would have to use those forbidden behaviors. School was the only emotional haven she had. Now she needed a physical out to compensate for the physical abuse she got at home. Her dream had been to earn a spot on the cheerleading squad. She soaked up status during those precious academic years. She worked extremely hard for months, practicing in her bedroom to gain enough confidence to perform in tryouts. She won a position on the squad. Cheerleading would now be her physical outlet.

Her smile dropped away giving her a serious expression. Barb began to doubt herself. *Maybe I'd just made up all that cheering shit? Maybe I was never a cheerleader.* Twisting to change her position caused a pain to flare in her lower back. Right then and there she knew it was the result of an old cheerleading stunt injury, thus completely validating her memories. She looked toward the heavens. *Thanks.*

In hindsight Barb was amazed at what she'd accomplished with cheerleading. Through all those years before high school, Barb had held on to her father's lies. She never once questioned him. *You are my special one,* her father used to say. He never wanted to share her with anyone or anything. As she got older he had to pull back on his control or he might have been caught. He was jealous of her independence during her high school time. To think that as a child she verbalized her allegiance to him, and in the process disowned and abandoned herself. She remembered being submissive to her father so that he wouldn't fly into a complete raging control trip. Through fear and threats of impending doom she always let him have his way.

"No! That's not true. It didn't happen that way. I…" Barb stopped his voice in her head in mid sentence. For once her mind fully opened, and for the first time she saw that her father used her as an object, a toy to terrorize for his enjoyment. He had programmed her with lies while she was very young. He had programmed her to believe she was bad, with no abilities, no talents, and no qualities. He had constantly berated and belittled her every move, thought, or feeling to keep her under his control. He made her repeat disparaging statements about herself for hours and forced her to pledge to him that she believed every word. He verbally tormented her by imitating her cries for help as he raped her. *Bitch. You made me do this to you!* He knew that if he couldn't control her and her tongue, he'd lose everything and be sent to jail for his crime.

Barb's father criticized every part of her body as not being good enough. *No one would ever want to look at your body. You're a homely bitch. Face it; you're homely.* He broke her down mentally and physically, making her feel small, worthless, and ugly. She remembered his getting a big boost to his self-esteem by harassing her. It seemed that the lower her self-esteem was the higher his became. Then she remembered something else. She had recalled asking her father once if she could be a cheerleader. He answered with one of his violent episodes. She had vowed then to do whatever it took to become a cheerleader. She would do it in secret, show him that she was pretty, smart, and wanted. Only the prettiest and most popular girls were voted onto the squad.

Momentarily drawn away from the black emotionally laden images of her father, Barb resisted being pulled into his distortions. Barb brought her mind back to happier times, her high school days, her time in the light, and her fifteen minutes of fame. She'd practiced for hours in front of the bedroom mirror everyday until just before her father came home. She had to have the movements down precisely, no mistakes. *Mistakes can kill you.* She practiced to exhaustion. Barb created a separate life behind her father's back. He would have beaten her bloody if he'd known how much effort she put into achieving her goal. *Bloody?* Barb thought. *Hell, he would have killed me.*

At the tryouts Barb was so nervous and fearful that she had to run into the girl's locker room to throw up between rounds. She rid herself of all anxieties once she started the routine. Her performance fooled the other contestants and coaches into thinking she had it all together. Against all odds she completed her routine flawlessly. She got up early the next morning and rushed to school to find out if she had avoided being cut. She was on the roster with the title "Invited to Join the Cheerleading

Squad." She had accomplished her goal. Full of happiness and pride, she had done it on her own.

Barb reflected on how she'd had healthy perceptions during that period of her life. Everything in the room stood still while a momentary sense of competence coursed through her body. She decided back then to keep her appointment to the squad a secret from the whole household. Her greatest accomplishment became her biggest secret. She couldn't tell her wonderful news to any member of the family because it would have gotten back to him. He would have flown into a rage and beat her for betraying him. She feared he would break her leg, thereby crushing her hopes and dreams for realizing her only chance to be in the spotlight. From that point on Barb led a fragmented life. She compartmentalized her cheerleading the way she pigeonholed the abuse. She acted one way at school, another way in front of the family, and yet another in front of her father. Barb's life was a juggling act of thoughts, feelings, and actions during those years.

Each cheerleading practice was a realization of her dream. Barb invested heart and soul in the squad. Her deep devotion and hard work drew attention from Coach Lee. A devoted friendship developed between them. Lee was the only one she ever trusted in school; maybe the only one she ever trusted anywhere. Barb gained much from the relationship. She went into the varsity squad as a freshman, an immature, shy, and somewhat overweight girl. Lee recognized talent and offered to tutor her. Together they built a strong, confident young woman. In her senior year she was elected captain of the squad. Coach Lee had seen her overcome many obstacles just to be a cheerleader. She took a sentimental breath and returned to reviewing her memories. Those precious years flew by so fast. Barb had been successful because of her ability to compartmentalize her lives. All the awards and certificates she won for cheerleading she kept in a shoebox deep in the farthest corner of her bedroom closet. Her honors went unrecognized by her family, her father, and sadly to say even by herself.

Images of that time continued to parade through Barb's mental vision. A sense of joy, pride, love but also deep sadness filled the empty emotional vaults of her heart. The parade of images included her biggest mistakes, some of the worst she ever made with her father. One night during her senior year near the end of the cheerleading season, she told him and the family about her involvement. Barb had naively thought he had changed and would be proud of her. He was openly tolerant of the news, but she heard an underlying current of violent rage in his voice, almost like a quiet growl. It was evident he didn't like her being on the squad, but he didn't openly express it with other family members present.

In that moment of memory, Barb thought maybe her father was jealous of her devotion to the squad. Or could it have been jealousy of the closeness he discovered between her and Coach Lee?

Over the years Barb had developed a denial mechanism to divert the pain of her father's never-ending rejections. She was his daughter, and he must have been proud. *Him, jealous? How could be jealous of the squad? That would mean he had emotions.* She laughed quietly in her thoughts.

Barb's breathing became rapid; her heart pounded. She caught herself and took a slow, deep breath and reasoned. *Hindsight is sometimes sickening. Hindsight, shit. Truth is sometimes sickening. Hell is a truth learned too late.* Reality punched her right between the eyes, clouding them with tears.

Barb continued reminiscing. Guilt began to creep up on her as she recalled her "blind faith" when it came to her father, her "perfect-father-thinking" that went on during that phase of her life. She rationalized that if he could only see her perform, he'd accept her accomplishments with as much pride as she felt. Again it was her falsely innocent perceptions that brought her dreams slamming to a halt. She finally convinced him to come to a game near the end of her senior year. She watched him get up and leave before the end of the third quarter. That night Barb received her worst beating. His evil words remain in her head.

You thought you were something, but you were nothing more than a slut out there! You embarrassed me in front of everyone in town, he said. The injuries he inflicted stopped her from going with the team to the state championships. She phoned the coach tell her she had fallen and couldn't perform. If Coach Lee saw the marks and bruises she would know. Barb couldn't afford that. It was easier to just remain loyal to her father and resign from the squad. She walked away from her dream to save *him*. The squad she helped develop, had invested in and nurtured went on to the state level without her. They won. At the pep rally, she sat alone in the bleachers and silently felt their happiness.

Tears invaded her eyes as she experienced true emotion. Her body jerked instinctively into a defensive posture because of the unfamiliarity of the sensation. Barb banged her head on the wall to purge the thoughts from her brain and return to the present. An electric stab of pain crackled through her body as payment for the indiscretion of remembering times of happiness.

Inside her mind under a cloak of self-imposed chaos, shame, abuser's values, and self-blame, hostile thoughts crept past her outer emotional defenses and fed off her pain and fear. Her attempt to halt such thoughts failed. *You never deserved any of that.* The pain continued to increase as her happiness faded.

The pictorial history moved to another benchmark in her life and dragged her emotions along. Barb viewed images of her first incident in a treatment facility, where her attitude toward her problems was one of arrogance and justification. She so needed to numb her pain that she had been drinking heavily for some time. Trying to think during those years had been like viewing a reflection in a broken mirror.

As soon as she began to contemplate that period of her life, she was mentally transported to a different era. Scenes from her first job came to mind. Her secret life as an abused wife had been discovered by the outside world. It all started to affect performance at work. Barb's periods of mentally "going away" had become too frequent and were recognized by her co-workers. She'd been summoned to the boss's office that black Thursday afternoon. Mr. Shamus stated that her job performance had decreased to such a level that he could no longer ignore the situation. It was causing problems with the other employees. She remembered the look in his eyes when he listed her options: "one, get help through the company's Employee Assistance Program, or two, quit." She felt so cornered and she seemed to separate from her body right in front of him. She remembered actually seeing herself frozen in that office chair as she looked down from the ceiling of the office. The female figure she saw in the chair appeared to be a mute three-year-old child who was scared and unable to debate the allegations flung at her.

Barb was more concerned about what her husband would do than about keeping her job. Surely he would beat her within an inch of her life if she were fired. The only way out of the situation was to go to the company's EAP. She visited the company counselor, and toward the end of the first session he recommended inpatient treatment for her alcohol addiction. Three days later she was in a recovery center. Withdrawal from alcohol proved to be worse than the pain she had attempted to drown.

Thinking about it brought a half smile to her face. It was at that first treatment center that Annie had become stronger and more apparent. It was Annie who was Barb's companion the entire time she'd been there. They spent endless hours together in Barb's head. Barb groomed Annie, giving her all the talents, characteristics, and qualities her first husband had been trying to exorcize. They deliberated on a method for replacing their lost faithful friend and servant – alcohol. Annie gained strength and became a protective resource for Barb.

While other members were disclosing secrets about themselves during one of the group therapy sessions, Annie and she devised a new numbing vehicle. The secrecy of their ongoing planning was what got her through the thirty days of treatment. Together they completely fooled the staff. Barb walked out one month later as a successful alumna. She returned to work an outwardly different person. Her ability to mask her pain became an art.

Shaking her head, Barb reexamined the days after she returned home. She had dried out while in treatment but never developed the ability to stay sober. She had to have some kind of mechanism to numb intrusive emotions and all the symptoms resulting from past abuse and trauma.

Exhausted from so much reflection, her body grew heavy, and she unconsciously drifted away into sleep. Aware of her transgression, she immediately shocked herself back to reality by pinching her right forearm with her fingernails. Confusion and helplessness surrounded her. At this point her ability to control the direction her mind was going failed and abuser's values charged at her again, flooding her with doubt.

An image of a small, lifeless room came into focus on her mind's screen. It was her childhood bedroom. Frightened, Barb assured herself it couldn't be. *It's not mine!* Tears streamed from her eyes, clouding her ability to see. *Oh, my God, it is; it's my parents' house. No, no it can't be. It is. It's my bedroom.* Her mind analyzed the scene as her body curled up protectively on the bed. Her reaction was one of fear, terror, and coldness.

Horrified and unable to cope with the flashing images, she coiled into an even tighter ball on the bed in the strange room. She had felt so alone and unsafe without Annie and with no way of numbing the constant pain. A flood of light abruptly invaded the room. In total fear she instantly opened her eyes to meet her attacker while making a tremendous mental effort to ground herself. *Oh, please stop. It's not happening now; it happened a long time ago. You're okay. Please stop.* Realizing where she was, she snapped back to alertness. *Don't move. Don't look suspicious,* she cautioned herself.

A shadowy figure broke the light by standing between her and its source in the hallway. Her first reaction was that a monster had come after her; then her eyes focused, and she identified the unit technician. "Are you all right?" the woman asked. Barb forced out a quick answer to avoid detection and pulled herself completely back into reality.

"Yes, I'm okay. I'm just a bit unsettled from the trip and lack of sleep. Thank you." Barb hoped she was convincing enough. For a second she thought she could pull off another "perfect patient" scam. She had done it before in other facilities. Staying vigilant, she lay quietly on the bed and listened for the technician's footsteps fading away down the hall.

Left alone again, Barb tried to shut off her thinking and go to sleep, but her mind returned to deeply stored memories which were searching for resolution. Images flashed on another admission to a treatment program. Four years ago she had to force herself into a food addiction facility. Barb had developed a sick obsession with food. Food became the only way she had to protect her innermost emotions through the constant beatings and sexual attacks by her second husband. Barb's obsessive alliance with food turned into an ugly, uncontrolled battle, and she lost. She admitted herself to a facility that specialized in treating that particular addiction. Annie came along for the experience. She was there for support and to help her plan on ways of getting through the treatment. Annie loved playing with the staff. Together they developed various games involving food. Barb learned more numbing techniques from her peers and graduated completely numbed out and more successful at hiding.

In Barb's thinking, food allowed her the only socially acceptable avenue for self-control. She told people when they remarked on her weight, "My whole family is skinny." She was caught between two opposites. Number one, she hated her body because of the mean things her father always said about it. Number two was that David hated her body if she showed any kind of weight increase. He made unreasonable demands that she maintain a slim, sexy shape. He perceived skinny as attractive. Barb went long periods without eating so she could fit into the embarrassing outfits David forced her to wear – clothes that made him fantasize, and got himself so excited that he'd rape her. Without warning he would brutally force her into performing many degrading acts. Her only emotional protection was to avoid eating. The anorexia allowed her to numb the pain, shame and guilt of what he did to her, yet such behaviors resulted in even more shame. She forcibly pushed her fingers down her throat to drive out the evil things David made her symbolically ingest. It was effective in eliminating the powerful sense of intrusion from her body, but the relief was only temporary. No one was aware of Barb's self-damaging course; even the ever-vigilant David didn't notice. He overlooked the harm her food problem caused and only admired the results. He didn't care what she had to do to fulfill his wishes as long as she did what he demanded. Mirrors became Barb's archenemies. Her mirrored self gradually faded over time until she no longer recognized the reflection that stared back at her – so she got rid of all the mirrors in the house.

Still unable to sleep, Barb's mind continued to search her forbidden memories. Food was a passive physical means of control, but it also represented self-punishment. Her repetitive, ritualistic avoidance of food became ingrained. Controlling food became as important to her as alcohol once was.

During the course of treatment for food addiction, Barb learned that forgoing alcohol was a simpler process than she had feared. The fight to let go of her abusing relationship with the bottle lost importance because of her new alliance with food. Rejecting any thoughts of her deep relationship with food, she willfully disconnected from her memories and finally fell asleep.

A loud knock startled Barb awake the next morning. Blinking to focus her eyes, she came to the shocking realization that she was in an unfamiliar environment. Confusion accompanied the wake-up call until reality reared its ugly head and her nocturnal fog vanished. *You're in a hospital. You will be all right,* she thought orientating herself to the unfamiliar environment. Her bones ached from the constant contraction of her muscles responding to her ever-operative vigilance. Her sensors remained alert even as she slept. She turned sharply toward the door as three sharp raps met its wood face for a second time.

"It's time to get up," commanded the unseen. Fear flowed through her veins at remembering she was in a treatment center. She was afraid of what the day would bring. She began to worry. *How should I act? How will the other patients react to me?* She slowly rose and dressed under the stress of enormous self-imposed fear. Although such feelings were strictly forbidden, she had a sense of wonderment, a rare excitement about things to come.

Waiting through breakfast for the first group session was excruciating. Barb was increasingly anxious and uncomfortable at meeting the other women to whom she had just become a peer. The actual group session found her mute and reserved.

Though the lesson for the day covered only the philosophy of the program, she found her thoughts in conflict. Here she was being told that people who survive trauma and abuse are powerful, creative, strong, and intelligent. Barb's previous experience with the helping profession taught that they perceived her kind of defectiveness as a form of attention seeking. Yet even with her defensive analytical ability, some of the principles made sense and opened her awareness. She was unwilling to trust the program, but she intended to challenge it by working as hard as she could. That way it would either work, or it was a lie just like the others. She was secretly afraid that she might actually possess some of the qualities they described.

    No matter what she learned in the daily groups, Barb held fast to the idea that she caused her abusers to perpetrate violent acts on her.

    From the left side of her brain, her father's voice chimed in to validate her current thoughts of self-blame. "You're right; all those times were your fault. You made me hurt you because you could never do things right. You did everything purposely to get me to do those things to you. Maybe I loved you too much." The voice silenced to allow the words to sink in and then continued. "Look around. You're not that bad. The other women here are worse than you. You don't deserve this! It isn't a crime just to love me. Get up and go home." A verbal harangue such as this was nothing new to her.

    Her father's voice didn't leave her alone for a single second, and he wouldn't let up on his running commentary. In the first week of treatment, she felt as torn as a turkey wishbone the day after Thanksgiving. Every day she fought with herself as to whether she should remain in the program and face her horrifying pain or leave out of obedience to her father, her addictions, or her symptoms. Her family had indoctrinated her to believe that membership in the family was a privilege that required absolute devotion. Her experience in treatment so far was in opposition to the argument in her head.

    What she was discovering in the program was that she had a hidden strength. Her inner energy and motivation increased with every group therapy session. Her thoughts remained confused but that didn't seem to stop her progress. As a result of the education, assignments, homework, and group experiences, she saw that she could learn, make decisions, and retain knowledge. She found that she wasn't broken, damaged, defective, dirty, or bad as she had been labeled by her father and husbands. Barb got stronger every day and began to learn why she was reactive emotionally and dedicated to her symptoms. She was getting healthier. A therapist taught her that what she did was a normal response to an abnormal situation, and anybody put in such circumstances at the same young age would have come out with similar symptoms but different symbols and behaviors. Barb had chuckled proudly to herself. *To think I was normal.* By using the skills she was learning, Barb began facing her fears without running or numbing. A seed of pride had begun to take hold within her.

One day in a moment of weakness during a therapy session, Barb reverted to her old negativity and started to compare herself to her peers. *They all get it and I don't. Why am I so different? I'm wrong. Am I too broken to make it through the program?*

Each group session helped to create more connections between her adult behaviors and symptoms and her childhood abuse. The more knowledge she gained the more armor she acquired. Barb began to correlate hidden emotions with her visual recollections. Yet all the intensive hard work she was doing in the program began to cause pressure and anxiety to mount inside her. To protect herself, she continued her old pattern of judging, analyzing, and interpreting everything inside and outside of herself. Keeping up with both exhausted her, and she was beginning to think she would emotionally explode or go truly insane. Her confusion and the conflict between her old life and the new information grew to such enormous proportions that fear took a back seat for a while.

After the therapists had left at night, the community of patients met on the patio for mutual support. Following an intense day of therapy the women shared wisdom with each other. Senior patients often spent the evening passing on the program's traditions and encouraging the newer patients. Some nights their only light was from a summer full moon. When she first came into the program Barb retired to her room and isolated herself doing homework rather than joining in with the others. After the first week her hunger for knowledge doubled. She felt more comfortable, socialized with her peers and participated more. During the evening discussions she soaked up all the information she could get. Though Barb's sleep patterns improved as she got stronger, a recurrent nightmare embraced her mind. Its realism demolished all attempts to ignore it. As soon as she passed into the depths of slumber, the same old images appeared. A view of a small girl in a familiar bedroom flashed onto her internal screen. The sound of claws tearing at a wooden door echoed in her mind. Filled with fear yet driven by an inner compulsion to discover what it was, the little girl climbed out of bed and tiptoed to the door. She placed her ear to the door's cold surface and heard a muffled growl. Trembling with fright, she reached for the doorknob.

Don't do that! It will kill you! she cried out in her sleep. But the child paid no attention to her anguished cry and slowly opened the door. A clear picture of deep scratches on the outside of the door formed in Barb's mind. The smell of wet fur filled her nostrils. Her mental vision swung 180 degrees to the right, meeting two fierce yellow eyes that peered back at her. Panic shook the little girl's frame from head to toe, and Barb shared her pain and fear.

Abruptly, Barb awoke shivering, sweating, and screaming for help. She huddled in a tight ball. The sound of rushing feet filled her ears. She saw a shadowy figure appear in the doorway to her room. It resembled the monster that had visited her when she was a child. She had difficulty telling if she had returned to the present or was frozen in her past of pain and hurt. The monstrous figure came toward her bed.

"What's happening? Are you okay?" asked her new friend, Beth, from across the hall.

"Don't touch me!" Barb screamed. Still not free of her dream, Barb raised her hands to shield herself from attack.

"You were having a nightmare," Beth said. "I heard you screaming from my room. I came to help." Barb explained her history of nightmares and the difficulty breaking away from them.

"I'm sorry I reacted that way."

"That's okay. You just need to use the tools they've taught us. What can you lose?" responded Beth.

By focusing and using her new skills, Barb was able to decrease her rapid breathing. Once that was under control her pulse rate returned to normal. She turned to Beth and spoke in a tone of camouflaged calm. "I'm all right now. You can go back to bed. Thanks you for coming to help. No one has ever cared like that before. Thank you."

"If you need someone, I'm across the hall. I'll be here for you." Convinced Barb was out of the woods, Beth returned to her own room.

Flopping onto her back, Barb stared at the ceiling until she saw the first light of morning. She continued to run the nightmare in her mind, looking for a clue, a message. Her efforts produced no meaningful answers. She was weak and exhausted from the nighttime skirmishes, but she imprinted the dream on her normal memory bank so she'd remember to ask the therapist for help in analyzing it. She was no longer shy about asking for help. She had learned in the program that the only stupid question is the one you don't ask.

She waited anxiously for Gooding the therapist to arrive on the unit. As soon as she did, Barb ran up to her and requested speaking time in the morning group. She paced the floor waiting for the start of the session, becoming more nervous with each passing moment.

The session finally started. "I have to tell you something," she said to the therapist. "I had a nightmare last night that frightened me a lot and I don't understand it. Please help me make some sense of it."

Barb described the experience while everyone listened without judgment or interruption. She stopped three times to loosen the knot that formed in her throat and went on to complete her story without any internal consequences. She rubbed the back of her neck to stop an oncoming headache as she searched the therapist's face for a response, an answer.

"What do you think it meant?" asked Gooding.

"I don't understand at all," she answered, as she lowered her head and scratched at its left side.

"Parts of your mind talk to each other in symbols during your sleep. Dreams are the process by which you resolve issues you haven't been able to cope with. They can be from your past or from today. A nightmare often carries a message you don't want to receive. Allow yourself to free your mind. Ask, could it have a meaning deeper than what I'm seeing?"

"I need some direction. I have no idea what else it could mean. Guide me please," replied Barb in frustration.

Gooding hesitated and pressed her fingers to her forehead before offering some direction in the form of questions. "Could your mind be telling you that the wolf is at your door? Could the wolf represent your fear and the door symbolize your well-armed defenses? Is it possible that you're afraid of knowing more about your life and yourself? Do you fear looking deeper because of what you might find? Or do you think you'll let yourself down again by betraying the promises you made to yourself? Could you be more scared of yourself than of what happened?" A puzzled look came across Barb's face.

"I'm still confused," she said.

"Then its working," said Gooding, who had designed her answer to help Barb feel rather than think.

Barb sat quietly, but her mind walked away from the group because of the therapist's remark. As Barb's focus faded from reality, the sound of Gooding's voice slid into the background and lost all importance.

If the answer is in me, then that's where I need to go. Barb sought further mental escape by fixing her gaze upon a corner of the molding on the window ledge. It helped her achieve a greater degree of dissociation to block out the possible overwhelming emotions. The window was in front of her and just over Gooding's shoulder. She was able to look right over her, hoping she wouldn't catch on to what she was doing. But the object – the molding

– she used for her cognitive release from the group backfired on her. Its shape triggered an unwanted response and transported her back in time. By studying the smoothness and shape of the wooden molding she was reminded of the basement window in her parents' house. She ignored the intrusive thought, trying hard to achieve a deeper level of numbness and find a way of not being sucked into her past. Her attempt failed. Her gut twisted into knots. She began to relive a memory, and in her mind it became real. This depth of knowledge had been forbidden to her in the past, yet somehow it felt familiar.

"Please Stop. Don't talk. Daddy will punish us again." Annie's barely distinguishable voice pleaded with Barb. "If you don't stop for yourself, then do it for me." But she couldn't distract Barb from her dissociative mission to numb out her painful feelings.

I must be dreaming. I must be inventing all of this, Barb thought. Doubt stampeded through her whole being while pictures flashed before her mind's eye. She withdrew her inner focus from the terrorizing images just long enough to scan the group members and measure her level of protection. She wondered if her peers recognized what was happening inside of her.

"Help me, don't abandon me again," Annie called from what seemed a great distance. It made Barb recoil inside her mind.

"Who's there? Is that you?"

"It's me," Annie replied.

Look, I've never left anyone. Everyone always left me first. Wasn't it you who left me days ago? Barb was shocked by what she heard in her head.

No answer came forth, so out of pure curiosity Barb returned her attention to the mounting images. A mental picture of a basement grew brighter and more frightening. Shame broke through her defenses and immobilized her. She instinctively closed her eyes, trying to short circuit her memory and stop the shower of pictures. The maneuver again blew up in her face. Shutting her eyes made the basement seem even more real and pulled her farther into it. Barb felt as if she were in that basement again. Her anchor to reality gave, and she began to slip ever further away.

Trapped in the memory, Barb shouted in desperation, *No, no I don't want to look. Oh, God, please help me. I promise to be a good girl. Stop it!* Tears of hopelessness streamed down her cheeks. Her nose registered a musty smell that lured her deeper into the basement. She caught sight of a small, tormented figure huddled in the darkest corner. When she'd identified that pathetic figure, fear rushed through her frail body. Gooding's voice broke into Barb's dissociative state.

"Open your eyes!" she suggested. "Open your eyes and look at me, please. You are safe. Just open your eyes and look at me. It happened, but it is not happening now. You do not have to relive it."

Barb made every effort to comply, but her eyelids seemed weighted and wouldn't open. Her throat constricted, so she couldn't speak. The feeling of being trapped was overpowering her defenses, and she began to panic. The therapist repeated her request in the form of a supportive command.

"Open your eyes. As long as they are closed, you're back there, and it's real to you. Open your eyes and look at me. It's all right. There's nothing here to hurt you. Seize reality and empower yourself; open your eyes." Gooding's voice sounded so far away. Barb felt as though she were in two places at once, split between reality and that smelly, terrifying basement. A weak little voice from the figure in the corner called to her for help. Barb was unable to respond to the insistent urging of the therapist, but she felt moved toward the small voice in her memory. Fear and danger lurked around Barb in the basement as she got closer to the child trapped down there.

Other group members joined the therapist in supporting Barb. Together they all encouraged her to open her eyes. A wave of warmth began to rise from the core of her being. She mentally squared her shoulders against her fear and began to chant silently, *I am not going there. I am not going there!* She desperately wanted to return to reality. Using every bit of strength she could muster, she tried to jerk her eyes open, but her eyelids seemed to be held shut by two powerful hands pushing on them.

Open, damn you, open. You can't stop me this time, Barb commanded. She tugged her facial muscles with all her might, and her lids flew open. As her vision cleared she found herself looking right into the face of the therapist.

"Keep looking at me, there's nothing out here that will hurt you. You have the power to stay here, change your position, breathe deeply, and use your strength to come all the way back to us," Gooding encouraged.

Realizing that her peers were gazing at her with concern, embarrassment swept over her. Exhausted from reliving the experience, Barb bashfully glanced around to see the reaction on their faces. She hoped that none of the group would display a negative reaction or be judgmental. *Well, at least no one is laughing at me.*

Barb was still trembling from the experience. Her lungs expanded to take in more oxygen. She glanced around the group once more. This time she saw expressions of true understanding. At that point Barb's feeling of aloneness began to dwindle, allowing her to reach a new level of self-awareness. At last she understood that she wasn't the only one who suffered the brutal effects of abuse and trauma. Barb validated her own normalcy. *They know. I'm not alone. I'm not the only one this ever happened to.*

"Are you back with us now?" Gooding asked.

"Yes," Barb answered as she swallowed against the fear that was again rising in her throat, but she continued speaking to the therapist. "I almost lost the battle. I had decided to face the terror head on this time and not surrender, but it sucked me in. I wasn't about to let it win, even though I was only reliving it. When I finally was able to open my eyes, my mind was clear about the difference between what happened then and what is now. I somehow knew I'd be safe here, so I fought against the hold it had on me." She paused for a moment to recover from her exhaustion. Inhaling deeply, Barb continued to address the group with her head held high. "This was the first time I beat it. I'm not as weak as they said I was. That was another lie they told me just to get me to keep their dirty secrets." Seeing that she had regained her balance, Gooding moved on with the group session.

Looking back, Barb understood it was the fastest she had ever recovered from such an intense dissociative episode. It used to take days, maybe even weeks of depression and emotional wrestling matches with shame and blame to release her from the clutches of her past. She also realized it was the strength emanating from the group members that gave her the courage to follow through.

When the session concluded, to her surprise, her peers asked if they could give her a hug. Barb had truly tasted her first success! She left the group with a sense of validation. Barb proudly but quietly said to herself as she walked down the hallway toward her bedroom. *You did it! You did it!* She actually took a little jump for joy and kept walking. Physically and emotionally exhausted by the time she got back to her room, she fell face down on the bed and passed out for a well-earned rest.

Startled out of a deep slumber, Barb strained to see in the darkness that encircled her. She sat straight up in bed, knowing she had been asleep for quite a while. *I must have slept all day and half into the night.* She was alone in her room while her peers were asleep. She monitored her pulse rate and blood pressure. Both were elevated. An unnatural presence surrounded her, and it seemed as if the room was being compressed. Sweat formed on her forehead. Enormous levels of pain paralyzed her limbs as chills raced through her already depleted body. A cloud formed over her, inhibiting her powers of judgment. Her father's voice cut through the silence with soft but stern authoritarianism. Barb sat up instantly.

"Bitch, you're still no good. You disobeyed me; you betrayed my wishes. You betrayed me. You must punish yourself for what you said. I told you not to talk about it."

I will not! Barb snapped back, horrified and overwhelmed. She remained active in reality by keeping her eyes open in order to gain new insight. She became painfully aware that she had gone through life seeing only what her father wanted her to see, not what really was there.

I won't do that; I haven't done anything wrong, she asserted.

"Hush now. You must honor my request. You love me don't you? Do it. Do it now," came her father's voice.

You think you're so damn smart and powerful. If that's true, then materialize. Come out here and punish me yourself. She felt as if she were facing a firing squad. Holding her chin up, she stared straight at the wall and waited.

Nothing happened, nothing at all. *You can no longer deprive me of my dignity. I won't allow it. I will not raise a hand to hurt myself ever again. You'll have to do it yourself, the way you used to.*

Barb braced again in anticipation of her father's fist. He always punched her in the face after she displayed even the slightest amount of boldness or insolence. She remained motionless, frozen in a defensive position, waiting for the monster, her father, to appear. She strained her eyes to see in the darkened room. Adjusting her hearing to the acute level, she monitored both her internal and external worlds. Not a sound could be heard. Without moving, Barb sat in her bed for the rest of the night, waiting for the first light of morning, prepared for the worst; but nothing happened.

In the morning she shared her latest nocturnal episode with the community, and was received with support and praise. Her newly acquired courage and developing skills had proven to be effective. It seemed as though her journey toward health had truly started. Barb wasn't always happy with the insight she found, yet she forged ahead. This morning she had successfully risked showing her inner self to others without acting out or engaging numbing behaviors. The events of the session, though successful, stimulated strong feelings of shame and self-blame; but she resisted them. Her just acquired strengths allowed her to appropriately reassign those negative accusations to her past abusers. *I don't need to be a misguidedly loyal person.* She understood that last night she had fought to keep the past out of the present, and she'd won. Barb also learned that she possessed a more-than-ample amount of strength, intelligence, and creativity to cope with life's everyday perils. The wisdom she attained through facing her "tunnel of pain" showed she did have power over her past. Barb envisioned her journey to recovery like going through a tunnel. At first approach it looked like an endless tube of darkness with no evidence of an end. Fear was her main emotion at that point, but she would pick up skills as she traveled. Toward the middle of the tunnel she was under constant attack emotionally and mentally; but she kept moving. She still experienced flashbacks and body memories, but thanks to learned skills, she felt like an observer of her past rather than a participant. Her commitment, faith, and determination to keep walking no matter what brought her to where she was now, the last part of the tunnel. Then she saw a small beam of white light visible in the distance. The farther Barb ventured toward it, the more the light expanded. Attacks were less frequent and less painful. She had new-found faith that the level of fear of her past would drop significantly. She had learned that if she just kept moving and looking forward toward the future, she'd reach the tunnel's end.

    With every skill Barb mastered she grew stronger. She learned that she was a person of value. Every day she rode an erratic cascade of emotions but held on successfully because she now understood that it was normal. Everyone's mood goes up and down during a day. *It is okay!* She told herself with pride. She renewed her commitment to making the process work for her. Her objective continued to be reconnecting with her body. *I want to feel like a normal person.* It was a phrase she had openly said all through her life.

    Day after day she grew in appreciation of her abilities and developed new values and definitions to live by. Her active involvement in the program earned a high level of respect from her peers. It was a feeling she didn't remember ever having except when she was a cheerleader. They helped her practice her new skills without judgment or criticism.

    One night as she sat in the shadows at the entrance to the hallway leading to the unit's sleeping area, Barb was startled by a noise. Out of the dark a friendly figure emerged. It was Gwen, a senior member of the group who was scheduled to reenter the outside world the next day. She sat down and engaged Barb in conversation.

"Been fencing, huh?"

"How did you know?" said Barb.

"I've been in the same state," Gwen replied.

"I've gone over it a million times in my head," Barb said, suddenly feeling shy.

"I know exactly where you are. I came to this program angrier and in greater denial than you did. I learned that my survival wasn't an act of weakness but an act of the heart. It was an undertaking of love to save me. As a result of abuse I had banished a part of me. Then for a long time I refused to accept any part of myself. I felt dirty, worthless, and hopeless. With the help of the program, I finally realized I was working against myself and serving my abusers. It was that part, which I now know I hid for safety, that I was always in conflict with. During sick times, I'd have done anything, and I do mean anything, for someone else; yet I wouldn't do anything for myself. My heart craved to be whole again, but I thought wholeness had to come from someone else and should happen automatically. If I loved someone enough, then I'd feel loved. No one ever told me I could do it for myself," Gwen said.

"How did you finally do it for yourself?" asked Barb.

"I asked to participate in the incorporation process," replied Gwen.

"So what was it like? Was it really helpful?" Barb asked.

"Incorporation allowed me to revisit my past safely and rescue that part of me I had hidden all those years. The most difficult part of the experience was to face and accept myself. I had trouble forgiving what I had hidden." Gwen paused in thought and let a small tear fall. "Let me put it this way: even if I'd had the opportunity to withdraw my decision, I'd still have gone through the incorporation process."

"Should I do it?" Barb asked.

"You have to answer that on your own," Gwen answered without hesitation. "Don't go through incorporation for anyone else. It's not a magic cure. Truly know why you want to do it.

The experience was a spiritual event for me. But be warned - the hardest part, recovery, comes after the incorporation. At that time I really wasn't aware of the level of commitment required. I heard and saw the improvement incorporation made with other ladies who were finishing up when I first was admitted. I don't think I was fully ready for the incredible amount of guts it takes. I focused on working for incorporation after that. I'd never had to take such responsibility. Everyone else used to tell me how to think, act, and feel. After I accepted what I thought was the forbidden part of me, I was fully responsible for my thoughts, behavior, and feelings. You have to reflect on the fact that incorporation won't be the end of your journey but only the beginning. Be sure you know what you're asking for; because you just might get it here."

"Does the pain ever end?" Barb bowed her head in momentary surrender.

"I always hoped for release from the shackles of my pain, but I wanted a quick fix. I wasn't willing to invest all my strength in a program. I held back some of my secret pains in case the treatment failed. I wasn't honest with staff members, and even less honest with myself. Until now no one in all those years could tell me how to stop the pain. To answer your question: be truthful with yourself. If you decide to incorporate, be ready to take total responsibility for self in all its aspects. I regained my personal power and noticed a change in how I thought, felt, and acted. I usually don't speak of such serious issues, but I've seen a true wanting in your eyes. Your journey will be hard and lengthy but worthwhile. Maybe the greatest discovery was my own wisdom," Gwen said.

"Please tell me more," Barb begged, looking for further answers.

Without warning Gwen stood up and looked deeply into her eyes. "Don't ask for something you don't want," she said, before melting back into the darkness from where she had come. Barb never saw Gwen again. Gwen was discharged from the program before breakfast the next morning.

Pondering the wisdom bestowed upon her, Barb remained in the hallway for hours without fear. Her mind danced with the pros and cons of moving forward on her journey to recovery or again surrendering her life to people who hurt her.

As the renewing light of morning washed into the courtyard, Barb saw her own face mirrored in the window in front of her. There was something new in her image that she had long been forbidden to acknowledge.

"I pledge I will not allow myself to return to a life of pain and misery," she declared aloud to her reflection. Thus she determined the future course of her life. She raised her skinny frame off the floor and readied herself to move on.

Chapter 4

Inner Journey

Days passed after Barb's encouraging encounter with Gwen. Her mental fitness continued to strengthen with every bit of information she gained from each group session. At night she concentrated on her homework. She had never liked schoolwork, but this was different. Her insight increased with each assignment to the extent that she didn't want to miss anything. It all helped her shift her focus from what had happened in the past to what she needed to do to attain her goals in the future. Her major accomplishment was the ability to feel healthy emotions, yet she knew that the act of simply feeling remained the weakest of her newly acquired skills.

Having made a brave decision, Barb signed the request form to be scheduled for an incorporation session. The prerequisite for undergoing incorporation was the ability to feel, and she had gotten there. She studied all the material in the workbook and interviewed many of the senior members on their ideas about incorporation. She watched closely when her peers experienced incorporation. Seeing positive results she finally decided. *I want to be incorporated no matter what it costs.*

Excitement danced through Barb's head the next morning in anticipation of the first group session. Today might be the day Gooding would deem her ready for incorporation. Her anxiety heightened at the mere thought of actually doing it. Though she was very excited, a strong message of doubt came from deep inside her mind. *Maybe I'm not good enough to be chosen.*

The concept of not being good enough was not unfamiliar. Barb's father had long ago planted the notion in her young mind. *I'm not good enough* was always lurking in the shadows to undermine almost every good thought she had. The inimical message waited patiently to strike anywhere, anytime. Just a hint of doubt was sufficient for it to infiltrate her thoughts, actions, and emotions. Her destruction was its goal.

"It's time for group," the patient in charge of roundup announced.

Barb went in and took her seat. Her head was down. When she looked up she saw one of the other therapists. Gooding was the one she needed and she hadn't arrived on the unit yet. Barb drifted into her thoughts expecting to be disappointed. But even with the "not good enough" message looming, she remained firm in her decision to recover. Reviewing her progress in the program, she was convinced that she had worked extremely hard and was sufficiently committed. She had searched her heart for the strength to let go of her symptoms and found it, successfully learning to take the power she had previously used to survive traumas and apply it toward recovery instead. During her journey, she had often contemplated leaving the program and recanting all secrets she had disclosed. *Leave, huh. Run is more the word,* she reflected. Barb was amazed at herself for staying in the program, beset with so much pressure and anxiety. But she had.

As a result of hard therapeutic work, Barb's mental boundaries had strengthened. To her surprise, they were doing a good job of holding back the enemy that lived within. She couldn't deny the reduced intensity of her flashbacks or the mastery she had attained using her symptom-management skills. For the first time in her life, she felt what others described as inner safety or mental peace. The program had offered her a safe place where she could at last face past horrors and pain.

Barb continued to reflect warmly on some of her other accomplishments in the program and went on drifting in thought. She pondered the struggle of a developing butterfly attempting to unfold from its chrysalis. She could empathize with that struggle. A strange sense of pride swept over her. Her immediate reaction was to think she had committed a wrongful act by indulging in prideful thoughts. She hesitated, waiting for repercussions. She then quickly checked her mental territory for incursions and found that her boundaries had held.

"So let's get started," the therapist said. The word we will work on today is loyalty. It's the most important word in your effort to recover. Misguided loyalty can stop your recovery at any point. Don't underestimate its enormous power."

Barb tuned out the lecture because she thought she already understood the point, and Gooding wasn't teaching it. She had developed a connection with Gooding and learned to respect her level of skill. She went back to mulling over the desired, no – hungered for – last piece of her puzzle, unification. She had learned how to revisit haunting images without reliving them. She had also faced her loyalty problem many times by using the Rapid Reduction Technique she had been taught. *At least I'll never have to relive my past again.* Calm rose from the core of her being. Decision made, she was committed to not turning back. She was prepared to embark on her journey into inner darkness to face self and to rescue what she had lost. If she was picked, she'd follow through with the incorporation. Once and for all she'd know whether she was really insane or not.

Over the weeks Barb heard from many of the senior members about their passage through the program. None would tell her any details of incorporation, but every one of them encouraged her to get connected emotionally before starting. They told her "All you have to do to recover is feel. Be honest and do the incorporation for yourself, alone, no one else. If she wasn't mentally committed she wouldn't accomplish her mission. Remember, feeling is healing."

The idea of feeling had been a foreign concept to Barb for all her life. Before coming to the program, feeling meant betrayal, something forbidden and painful. She would do or take anything in order to numb out all feelings. Yet after thirteen days in the program, she now embraced the concept of healthy feeling, and it was slowly becoming a way of life. The idea of continuing to work at reconnecting her emotions with her thinking was now attractive to her. The act of fusing her head to her body to feel was still a concept foreign to her. She had always seen things in black and white. She felt as if she had been walking a tightrope in her nearly two weeks of treatment. Memories of terrorizing nights in her childhood, days full of gut-wrenching pain, and her need to demonstrate strong loyalty to her father were now growing faint. Yet her father's haunting voice remained ever present, and she knew he was still monitoring her movements, thoughts, and emotions.

Barb had gained enough skill to enter her memories without numbing her emotions, free from fear, and without an escape plan. She had achieved a level of comfort and felt safe enough to look within herself, even in the presence of her peers.

Her elbow registered a jostling that brought her thoughts back to the present. Irritated by the interruption, Barb turned to chastise the other group member. She stopped cold because of the display of excitement on the woman's face. She was nodding her head toward the door and whispering, "It's your turn."

"What?"

"Gooding wants you. She's pointing at you. Good Luck."

In disbelief Barb apprehensively turned her eyes toward Gooding, who was peering at her through the open group room door. Pointing at Barb, Gooding beckoned for her to follow. In surprise Barb pointed at her own chest and mouthed the word "me?" Gooding nodded, and Barb rose from her chair and slowly moved toward the door. She stopped, turned to the others and winked. As she neared the door, blood drained from her head, and her anxiety increased with each step, leaving her both excited and afraid. Barb knew in that instant that the time had really come; there was no turning back. The arduous trip to Gooding's office began. Her protective vigilance system came on line and was operating in high gear. All senses activated, she kept walking. If she didn't keep moving she knew she would feel trapped and collapse in the hallway before making it to the office.

Barb fell back as Gooding picked up her pace. All her energy was directed toward not letting on that she was having trouble controlling herself. *Am I afraid or excited?* She couldn't allow Gooding to discover any imperfection or weakness in her resolve at this point. If she perceived that Barb wasn't ready, she'd return her to the group. She couldn't tolerate such a significant setback.

"Don't do it! I've warned you! Stop before you make the ultimate mistake!" Her father's voice rang in her head. "Don't betray me any more! Everything can be forgiven. I can fix it all. Please don't do this." Experiencing great discomfort, Barb ignored her father's voice, locked her eyes on Gooding, and just kept walking. Only one more hurdle stood between her and the wholeness she had been working so hard to achieve.

I can do this, she thought, cheering herself on. *There's only one last step to go. Seeing my truth can't be as bad as the torture I've gone through all my life.* To reduce the mental chatter, she began repeating, *I am worth it for me. I am worth it for me. I am worth it for me.*

Her father's harsh voice pushed its way through her chanting. "You'll die if you see. You don't want to witness all that. Stop! I warn you that I can still get to you." She tried to ignore his verbal intimidation but this time felt a stinging pain at the base of her skull. "See, I can get to you. If you do not stop what you are doing I'll kill you. This madness will not go any further," her father's voice threatened.

Barb's inner torment continued to flare up, and her anxiety grew. She tilted her head back as though she were looking up at her father. *I will never get better if I don't look.* The paternal voice changed its tune.

"That program has just filled your head with shit! Good girls don't tell. Everything will change, I promise. You are my princess. Don't abandon me." His words cut through her like a scalpel. Not concentrating on where she was walking, Barb ran right into the figure standing in her path. Gooding turned around, looked into her eyes, and spoke with compassion.

"I know you're scared. You're probably being threatened in your head right this moment. I understand that you feel like this is a severe betrayal, but you deserve a life. Gooding opened a rather ordinary looking door and motioned Barb inside her office. She proceeded with extreme caution. She was still debating whether she was afraid or tense with excitement. She felt a sudden pressure on her chest as though an unfriendly hand were pushing her backward. She stumbled but caught her balance and straightened up without drawing suspicion.

Gooding directed her to the blue-green recliner placed against the opposite wall. Barb went over and sat down. Her hands were turning cold and clammy, and she could hear her heart pounding in her ears. The therapist hung a big butterfly flag on the outside of her office door and closed it. This told everyone that an incorporation session was in progress, and there could be no interruptions. Gooding pulled a straight-backed chair to the left side of the recliner and settled in. Crossing one leg over the other she gazed intently into Barb's brown eyes. "Anxious?"

"Yes."

"Good. It is very normal and the best vehicle." Gooding chuckled. A long pause ensued. She looked Barb straight in the eyes and asked, "Are you ready?"

"I am"

Gooding got up and moved around her office, gathering papers and reducing the light. Then she sat back down, "Do you really want to do this?" she asked.

"I do."

Both of Barb's worlds, internal and external, were actively clashing at this point. She had to fight to cover up the barrage of emotions emanating from them. Her boundaries were holding, but not without a price. Barb didn't want Gooding to uncover her mental chaos. She feared that if she recognized her emotional conflict, she would deem her not ready. Her ability to hide such conflict had always been successful, but this woman was different; she could "see." A rush of anxiety flooded her senses. Discovery had long been a terrible fear as it had always been followed by punishment.

The program had given Barb the ability to feel, but now it seemed to be working against her. For a fleeting moment she doubted that her decision to incorporate had been the right one. She quickly shook off the feeling.

Gooding didn't appear to notice her difficulty. She was preoccupied with gathering the material she needed.

"Bitch. You bitch." Out of the blue she heard Annie's frightened scream within her. "You've gone too far! Stop now! I order you. I will not be a party to this! You've understood from the first what he could and would do to us. If you go through with this act it will be the end of us. Give up the secret and the threats will come true!" Annie had always understood the penalty for betrayal – their body would be killed.

It's my last chance for life, or we're dead for sure, Barb replied.

Discounting Barb's statement, Annie continued to speak. "I've been here for you all this time. I took all those beatings for you from Daddy. I've had to be with your repulsive husbands while you were gone. I did my best. You owe me." Silence invaded the moment while Annie got her wind. "This is the way you repay me? I deserve more than death."

Barb plead her case. *I cannot take the pain any longer. My life hasn't been a life at all; it's been a prison sentence. Hell! Prison would have been a resort, it was more like slavery. That's not living. Recovering is for both of us, not just for me. We are one and the same. I have come to terms with how I used you to escape the realization of what our father was doing to me. I developed you to shield me against that reality. I'm sorry, but I had no choice. Help me complete this task.* Barb hoped Annie would consider her final and strongest message.

Barb didn't wait for an answer. If she continued the conversation in her head, Gooding would recognize what she was doing. Another burst of pain from an unknown source and she began to slip away from reality, loosing track of time and space. Gravity seemed to press down on her, trapping her in the chair and making movement impossible. Her body withstood wave after wave of excruciating pain, almost to the point of letting it pull her out of the moment and sabotaging her chance of recovery. She prayed for the strength to ward off a breakdown.

Sensing the invisible physical restraint, her father's voice reached from far within her mind. "I told you! You can never escape my reach."

Barb's toes gripped the inside of her shoes. She had to maintain a sense of reality. She sent a command to her mind: *This is not the time to surrender! Keep brave! Stay present!*

On the verge of collapse and concerned for her safety, she visually reconnected and immediately began to scan the room. She redirected her thinking by familiarizing herself with the office.

Since she was about to grant entrance into her mental space, she searched for clues to help her better understand Gooding. Information gained from the décor didn't seem to match Gooding, as Barb knew her. Stuffed animals, pictures, and piles of papers reflected a softer, caring side of the therapist who was known to the community as the "seer." Data compiled from her scan revealed she was a contradiction in terms – just like herself.

Gooding sat in the chair on Barb's right and began questioning her once more. "Do you understand that incorporation could change your whole life?"

"I'm willing to risk it as I can't live the way I have been living any longer." Barb swallowed hard, "I have to know what really happened. It's the only avenue left that might grant me access to my childhood. I've always felt that a piece of me left and hasn't returned. I need to attempt incorporation for my sanity."

"Incorporation is not a way to recover or validate trauma memories. The incorporation process isn't without its consequences, both positive and negative," Gooding warned. She leaned toward Barb, connecting visually. "Incorporation is about finding self, and taking back what you lost."

Barb's emotional monitors suddenly registered intimidation. Keeping an eye on Gooding, she understood the other woman wasn't the source of her menaced feelings. She realized they were not alone. Her senses told her someone dangerous was standing right behind her. Barb nonchalantly looked around, making a visual check. It revealed no one there, nevertheless her anxiety increased with feelings of being threatened. Betrayed by anxiety, her left leg began to bounce rhythmically.

So many abrupt internal changes caused a single tear to trickle down Barb's cheek. Fear invaded her senses. She hunted for an object to focus on so she could disconnect from reality. She needed to dissociate by moving into her sacred territory without letting the therapist know what she was doing. But Gooding picked up on her ploy and confronted her. "Where are you going?" Barb spontaneously returned to the present and rebuffed the question.

"Nowhere, I was thinking about your last question." Barb hoped she would accept the answer. Gooding looked her straight in the eye. "I need you present so I can help you get what you want." Then she scratched some notes on a pad.

Barb's usually reliable escape window had just been slammed shut. The only avenues open to her for help were her own skills and cooperating with the therapist.

"What do you remember?" Gooding continued her questioning with no hesitation.

"I remember nothing before the age of eleven."

The all-powerful voice of her father shoved another message at her. "That woman doesn't need to know anything about our relationship. It's our secret. You've always been my special little girl. You're just like me. I'll change for you! I promise."

A creepy silence took over the room while Barb thought about the voice and not the message. An image of her father's stern face flashed through her mind. *Oh, that can't be true! I'm nothing like him.*

"Whom are you listening to? Gooding confronted her again. What is the voice in your head telling you?" Gooding paused but looked at her very intently. "Not to give me any information?"

"What made you think that?" Barb mumbled in surprise. Tears filled her eyes when the base of her neck suffered another sharp pain, another warning signal. She was growing weaker from all the internal strife.

"Don't tell this asshole anything. Good girls don't betray their fathers!" He said trying to block her thoughts. Overpowered by a rush of intense devotion, Barb gasped for air and tightly pressed her lips together. She was stunned by the power of the silent exchange with her parental enemy. Afraid, she once more attempted to slip away into her sacred place but consciously stopped, thinking she might get caught out again.

Annie, help me! I'm frightened. Please, I am sorry for what I said to you. I don't think I can continue with Father berating me. I need you! she begged in mental darkness.

Waiting for Annie's reply, She ignored Gooding's voice. Her listening devices scanned at maximum level but heard nothing. The burden of sadness, loneliness, and abandonment was unbearable.

Slow cruel laughter rolled through the depths of her mind. Her father's angry voice broke in. "She won't help you anymore. You'll have to deal with me if you continue. Stop this insanity immediately."

In an effort to remain present, Barb forced the nails of her left hand into its palm. *I'll face it myself*, she said. Instinctively knowing the struggle Barb was having, Gooding leaned forward.

"It's just a taped voice in your head. It can't hurt you. It can't come out and hurt you. It's been active for so many years in your mind that it truly feels as though it's real and alive, but it's not. Gooding leaned back in the chair and placing a finger on her right temple asked Barb a straightforward question. "Do you really want to get better?" The intensity in the air doubled.

"Yes I do! I haven't worked this hard to just give up now." She exclaimed looking Gooding right in the eyes.

"Then understand that the voice in your head has one job and one job only: that is to make sure you don't tell its secret. It will say anything or cause you physical pain to keep you quiet. Loyalty to the secret is its objective."

Barb's face showed fear.

"Do you want to stop or go forward? It's your choice," Gooding said.

With that one question Barb's life hung on a thread. Her level of anxiety grew at the speed of sound. If she let the opportunity to incorporate slip by, she might never get another chance, and she would surely die.

"I want to go forward," she replied with confidence.

Silent and deep in thought, Gooding pondered Barb's fate. This moment of silence increased Barb's anxiety as she assumed that the therapist was disappointed or upset with her answer.

Gooding began again. "I will ask you three questions, and depending on your answers I'll decide whether to move forward or stop." She paused to write on the pad in her lap.

"Why do you want incorporation?"

"I want to live. I can't deny what happened any more. I want to get back what I was forced to leave behind," answered Barb.

"What is your biggest fear about doing the incorporation?"

"I am afraid it won't work for me, or I'll get inside and not be able to return."

Gooding nodded and asked the third and final question. "Without giving any details, noting only the general categories, what types of abuse do you know you have experienced?"

Barb sat in frozen silence and just stared at her until she repeated the question.

"I have suffered physical, sexual, emotional, verbal, and confinement abuse." As soon as she uttered the last betraying word, Barb felt a mental shift that seemed familiar to her but being under the watchful eyes of the therapist, she didn't have time to consider it. She felt an increase of alertness and strength, yet seemed comfortable and relaxed. With awareness now more acute, Barb sensed Gooding's eyes once more locking on hers.

"Are you ready to do some work?"

Barb nodded, and before she could reconsider, Gooding directed her to close her eyes, take three deep breaths, and affix a dot on the inside of her forehead between her eyebrows. She instructed Barb to focus on the dot until Gooding told her to disconnect from it. With each breath, she went mentally deeper into herself, clearer in thought and stronger in spirit.

"I want you to construct a platform in the back of your mind," the therapist continued in a soft monotone. "You can build it any way you want out of any material you want. Tell me when you're through."

"Don't do this. You don't want to go there. Stop while you can. I thought you loved me," came her father's voice.

Barb's thinking seemed split in half. One part was working to construct the platform while the other part attempted to deal with the idea that her father's evilness was monitoring her every move toward wellness. Despite feeling panicky, she was able to complete construction of the platform.

"It's done," Barb stated, recommitting herself to continuing the journey.

"I want you to mentally place yourself on that platform, but not until I say so. If you're successful, a staircase will appear at the other end of the platform. It will be illuminated, safe, and protective. The staircase leads down from your platform, through your head, neck, upper body, lower body, and all the way to your toes. Do you understand?" asked Gooding.

"I do."

"At every fourth step on the staircase there will be a corresponding platform to your left." Once again her father's critical voice attempted to interrupt Gooding's instructions.

"I'm warning you, you little bitch. You don't want to see what's down there. You won't be able to cope with it. You meant everything to me. Don't betray me."

Barb tightened her facial muscles, trying to minimize her father's torturing voice. She had to respond to her father's statements without getting discovered by Gooding. *You can't stop me this time. I protected you all these years and for what? What did it get me - love, nurturing, or punishment? Nothing but Punishment. I can't continue to live with your secrets. The pain and the price are too much for me to bear any longer. You've blinded me and kept me in the dark. You separated me from other people, the rest of the family, the world, and especially myself. Now it's my time to see. I want back what you took from me.*

Pretending to be unaware of Barb's conflict, Gooding went on giving guidance and instructions. "At the end of the platforms there may or may not be an image, a symbol or a memory of past pain. If you do connect with one you'll be able to revisit it safely rather than having to relive the pain. Do you understand?"

"I do."

Barb concentrated on Gooding's words. At that point she totally accepted the therapist's guidance and relaxed her guard. She was growing stronger and paying less attention to her father's voice, though he wouldn't give up trying to stop her. Her body eased into another level of comfort. She was about to descend into self, but this time she felt right about the mission. Fear and apprehension had diminished.

Mentally confirming that she was standing on the platform she built, Barb looked down at her feet and saw them pointing toward a staircase at the other end. She was ecstatic that she had made it through the first part and hadn't died.

"Now I want you to walk over to the top of the staircase. Let me know as soon as you are there" Gooding directed.

Barb gasped for air when a lump suddenly formed in her throat. *This isn't real. He isn't choking me. More of his tricks. He isn't here. Center. Focus.* She almost panicked into opening her eyes, thus signaling to Gooding that she wanted to terminate the procedure. But a light went on in her brain. *I get it you want me to stop, right? You want me to run.* She had figured out that the constriction in her throat was a ploy to divert her thoughts from her immediate objective – symbolic movement toward the staircase and her ultimate goal of wholeness. It was a mental instrument of her evil father's design. He wanted her to renounce her determination and assume a loyalty role. Barb was about to enter the forbidden area when there appeared an image of her father's large hands choking her. *Great graphics*, she quipped mentally. Refocusing, she transported herself to the top of the staircase, and for the first time confidently awaited further instructions.

"I am there," she reported. She now understood something her peers had reported about incorporation. She quickly referenced what they had told her. During their incorporation sessions they had an acute awareness of being on a "self" journey, acceptance of self, consciously, in reality, and firmly attuned to their emotions.

"When I tell you and not before then, I want you to walk down the stairs one step at a time, taking as many steps as I say.

Do you understand?" Gooding offered her an opportunity to take a risk. "If you agree, I want you to walk down the first four steps and let me know when you've done that. Do you understand?"

"I do."

"Go ahead now,' Gooding said.

Barb took a deep breath and in her mind and stepped off the platform. Her pulse quickened to twice its normal rate. *Step one,* she thought. Barb's acutely attuned senses remained at full alert for another attack. She counted until she reached the fourth step and stopped. She panned across the scene, saw an opening, and discovered that Gooding was telling the truth. There was another platform to her left. Standing on the fourth step, fully conscious and alert, she reported, "I'm there." Gooding gave some last minute instructions.

"From this point on you will revisit but you will not relive any painful images or memories you may come in contact with. You'll observe your pain, not reexperience it. You will be able to describe whatever you experience mentally or emotionally. Don't analyze, interpret, or judge anything you see, think, or feel. Just describe what you see at the end of the platform. I won't leave your side. I will be right here with you by your side until your journey is complete." Gooding paused a moment. "Now turn to your left in your mind and walk out to the end of the platform. Tell me what you see."

Barb did so, but fearfully. She couldn't raise her head to look off the end of the platform into the darkness.

Too much time had elapsed, so Gooding spoke. "Describe to me what you see!"

"Nothing," she said.

"Go on, just describe to me what you see."

"Okay, all I see is blackness," Barb replied in a voice devoid of emotion. She bit down on her tongue too afraid to look. Familiar feelings of small-girl helplessness returned. She kept her eyes tightly shut so as not to see what had really happened. She felt so childish and frightened standing there on the platform. A surge of loyalty assaulted her and she again began to doubt whether her decision to incorporate was right. *Do I truly want to know? Do I dare risk it?* Barbs attention was jerked around by a verbal attack from behind her at the top of the staircase.

"I told you so! I knew you couldn't betray me. You're a good little girl!" Her father's voice chuckled with enjoyment.

Barb momentarily lost all her strength and resolve. Doubt rolled over her like a blanket of fog. Without resistance, confusion marched past her entrenched defenses making her question her inner journey even more. *Am I just defective? So much different from the woman who incorporated before me? What did I do that was so wrong?* Regaining her power and stopping the ever increasing cycle of doubt, she shouted *I am not your little girl any longer and I won't be controlled!* With that she bravely opened her mind's eye. She looked straight ahead and reported to the therapist, "all I see is darkness."

Gooding saw the resistance and fear on her face but didn't allow her to sabotage her journey. "Return to the staircase, turn left, and walk down twelve more steps. Nothing can stop you from getting where you want to go. Let me know as soon as you're there."

Gooding's objective was to get her to refocus on her mental journey. Self-forgiveness could occur at any level. Experience told Gooding Barb's reaction was a common one. Her ultimate clinical mission was to assist Barb in rescuing the core self that she had hidden and left so long ago.

Gooding encouraged Barb to continue deeper into her internal matrix. From experience of conducting hundreds of incorporations, Gooding knew she didn't have to uncover every lost image to validate her pain and rescue her "self". She used a pattern of odd and even numbered platforms because some people view images on one and not the other.

Barb forged ahead down the staircase, but a cold sense of panic overtook her as she reached the twelfth step. She stood there with the fourth platform to her left and waited to see what came next. Gooding repeated her earlier instructions.

"Remember, from this point on you will revisit, but not relive anything that you may come in contact with. You will observe your pain, not reexperience it, and you will be able to describe whatever you encounter. Don't analyze, interpret, or judge anything you see, think, or feel. Tell me what you see at the end of the platform. I'll remain with you until your journey is complete. Now turn to the left in your mind and walk out to the end of the platform."

The fog of doubt lifted as quickly as it had come, and Barb's thinking became crystal clear. *Talk is cheap!* She challenged herself. *This time look! You're the one who decided to follow through with incorporation, so finish what you started. He can't hurt you any longer.*

At that instant her mental screen opened, letting an emotionally packed image dart across it. Its intensity fizzed like electricity all around her, yet she felt surprisingly protected and encapsulated in a cocoon of warmth. She was viewing an image that took her back to a traumatic incident that had negatively shaped her life. Oh, yes, the incorporation process had its penalties and consequences. Emotions steadily crept through her body and threatened to swamp her. She stood her ground. If that wasn't enough, her father's pleading voice came from what seemed to be the top of the staircase, "Please don't. I beg you. Don't go any further, please."

Hang in there and focus on what's important, she reassured herself.

"Describe what you see," Gooding requested calmly, breaking into her thought process.

"I see a house," Barb said after taking a deep breath. She hesitated to examine the image more closely. "It's the house where we lived when I was three years old." A single tear fell from the corner of her left eye. "Someone's coming out the front door. It's my mother. She's leaving for her job." Sounding sorrowful, Barb continued, "She did the best she could. My dad always demanded that she work, especially on the night shift. He said someone always must be home with me. Mom had no idea what he did to me while she was away. He treated all of us kids like prisoners." Her body jerked from a sudden pain in her lower back. She ignored it as just another attempt to throw her off and kept looking at the image.

"I know where I am!" she said with excitement. She mentally zipped though the rooms of the house. The back pain increased, almost causing her to seize up mentally, but she pushed on. She came to her second-floor bedroom. "There I am," she blurted out.

"Damn it, turn around and leave! Don't look! I command you!" A weaker parental voice reached her. For a split second it seemed as if a hand grabbed her heart. A spontaneous upsurge of strength from her inner core enabled her to confirm that she wouldn't die if she continued to face the pain. Ignoring her father's threatening orders, she pressed on. *Hang in there. You have a right to see the proof that everything he ever told you was a lie.*

"Run the images all the way through until they stop and continue to describe to me what happens," Gooding interjected. With her chin held high, Barb began to report. "I can make out a shadowy little figure huddled in a corner of the bedroom. It's me at three years old, and I look afraid. Now something's blocking me from seeing her clearly." Physical reactions to fear pulsed through Barb's body. Her heart was pumping. Alarmed at its increase, Barb paused. Gooding saw her stiffen.

Silence fell over the office while her systems rapidly examined the situation and reported. Her mouth began to move, but no words came. Her face contorted with the effort to speak. "I'm seeing my first bedroom. Oh, dear God! Don't let what I see be true."

Awareness confirmed her worst expectations, but she managed to speak to the therapist. "That little girl in the corner is me. My father is in there too, and he's hurting me. Oh no, please God no." A cloak of secrecy draped itself over her rigid form, followed by the sensation of her father's fingers closing around her neck. Again his deep voice angrily pleaded with her not to continue. With great courage she went on describing the scene, "The little girl is afraid. He's going into a rage." Gooding watched Barb cringing as if trying to protect her head.

"I always thought I was hurt by a monster but it was my father. He has a stick in his hand. He's hitting her, punching, and screaming names at her. Stop this pain." Panic began a stampede through every part of her.

"Freeze that picture now," Gooding instructed her. "Move your position until you can see the little girl's face."

"Okay! It's frozen. I'm where I can see her face," she stated between gasps.

"From what you have observed, did the child ask for this to happen?" Gooding queried. "Did she cause it to happen?"

"No, she wasn't doing anything wrong. She was just playing in her bedroom."

"Did it happen because she was bad, broken, defective or damaged?" Gooding asked. Barb studied the innocent figure closely.

No, she looks healthy.

"I want you to remember that. Now let the images continue to run until they end, but you can speed it up as fast as you want. Let me know when it stops. You don't have to watch it."

Regaining her composure, Barb drew a slow breath and did as Gooding asked. She chose not to speed up the images, but to witness what she couldn't have borne many years ago. Her report went on. "He's yelling at her, but she doesn't know why. What made him do it?"

"Turn up your hearing and report what he's saying to the child,"

"He's calling her a slut, just like her mother. She will never be good for anything or anyone. No one will be able to tolerate her; no man will ever want her," she intoned. The mental pictures kept coming, graphically depicting scenes of sexual manipulation and physical torture.

"He's tying her hands and feet together," Barb reported. "Oh, no, he's ripping her nightgown open, and cutting her chest. She's bleeding. He's moving away."

"Don't take your eyes off the little girl. Do not look at the act," Gooding ordered.

"He's coming back!" Barb screamed in fear. "Why won't he stop? He has a piece of metal pipe. God, he's beating her arms with it." Anger and horror roughened her voice. "He's saying,

I'll teach you a lesson, you worthless piece of shit. No one will ever want you after I get done with you. You won't ever leave me. I own you.'" An expression of shock appeared on Barb's face as she went on with her description. "Oh, he's really angry. He's dragging the little girl from the bed to the closet. I can't see. His body is covering what he's doing to her. He has tied her to the hook on the back of the closet door, and she's just hanging there. It's sick. He's closing the door so no light can reach her. He's saying vicious things, and she can't take any more. I can't continue watching." She paused to recoup and returned to listening. "You'll remain hanging there until the evil runs out of you. One word and you'll make me do something you'll regret." He closed the door, leaving her separated from the light.

"You have to continue till it stops," Gooding instructed. "Speed it up if it hurts too much. Let me know when it's over."

"I can't do it any more!"

"Freeze the image. Why can't you finish?"

"It's my father."

"Do you want to stop the incorporation?" Gooding asked with great empathy.

"No I want to continue. I have to finish," Barb pleaded.

"Then don't look at him. I want you to fix your vision on the child."

Barb repositioned her point of view, unfroze the image, and did as Gooding asked, but she was still reacting to what she had just learned. She accelerated the images. The therapist's words served to stop her from analyzing what she had just witnessed. Barb froze the picture at the end. Freed from the grip of intense anguish, she frantically replenished the air in her lungs. A sense of comfort surrounded her as the tense muscles in her back eased. She waited a second to rest.

"He was a sick man!" Barb commented with burgeoning self-confidence. Now that her memory was clear about that particular incident, she could understand why she always thought of herself as being broken, flawed, defective, and worthless. She began to blurt out harsh judgments about herself. "I can't believe I left her there with him," she paused to reflect, trying to rationalize what she had done. "I thought I was about to die. I didn't know what to do, so I left the only way I knew how – through my mind. I wanted to live and had to save what I could. His sickness was frightening; I left her there, and lost her there. I feel so ashamed. I now know why I hated me."

"Have the images stopped?" Gooding inquired.

"Yes."

"When I tell you I want you to reverse the image back to the beginning until you can see the little girl alone in the bedroom before the events started and then freeze it again. Do it now."

"Okay, I'm there. I see her," she announced.

"Now, in your mind walk off the platform. You will be supported and safe. Go into that image, pick up that three-year-old in your arms, and bring her back to the platform. No one can stop you or hurt you while you're in the image. Tell me when you're back on the platform with her."

Barb quickly moved into the image. When she scooped up the child huddled in the corner, the little girl rested her head on Barb's chest and felt the comforting warmth of her embrace. All the hurt melted away like icicles on the first day of spring. Barb sensed a level of peacefulness she had never known. She gazed into the little girl's innocent eyes, knowing they were a part of each other. Hurrying out of the image to avoid capture by her father's image, she ran back to the platform. "We are there," she stated.

Gooding instructed Barb to remain on the platform so she could communicate her feelings of forgiveness and acceptance to the sweet child she held.

"Repeat these words out loud after me," Gooding said. Barb agreed. "I'm sorry I had to leave you, but that's the only way I could survive. I thought I was facing death. What I learned since then is that I can't live without you, so I've returned today to rescue you. All the shame, blame, and guilt was too great for me to handle, but now you can return and live with me so I can become whole – happy, and healthy, free and safe. I will be protective, confident, and successful from this time forward. My illness was not my fault. You or I did not cause him to do those horrible acts. If you return with me I promise never to judge you, dismiss you, abandon you, or reject you ever again. I truly love you." Gooding observed Barb's physical reaction to her declaration and the influx of intense emotion.

"Repeat after me," Gooding started again. "I have to leave you for a few minutes to go forward in my journey. You'll be safe on this platform, and I promise I'll be back soon. When I return I'll never, ever leave you alone again." She issued more instructions: "Give her a hug then put her down on the platform." She paused to give Barb some reassurance, "I promise we'll come back for her." Gooding let her statement reinforce Barb's sense of safety. "Are you ready to go on?" She asked.

"I am."

"Then turn around in your mind and walk back to the staircase. Let me know when you're there."

For the first time since approaching the first platform, she stopped, and resisted Gooding's directions. The idea of leaving the little child, even for a second, wasn't right. Deep sadness and a feeling of abandonment took center stage in her heart. She stared with love at the little girl, afraid to let her go.

"It's okay," Gooding said, "she'll be safe on the platform until we return, no one can hurt her." Barb's frozen expression began to soften. "I'm back at the staircase." she said.

"Good! Now turn left and descend twenty more steps. Let me know when you reach the twentieth one." Gooding saw her face grow more frightened as she moved down the stairs.

Thoughts came darting up from the deepest reaches of Barb's mind. As she drew to the twentieth step, a dark shadow covered the staircase. She continued and found out that she could step right through it. She closed her eyes, lowered her left leg to the next step and put her weight on it. When nothing bad happened she kept on descending, one step after another.

"I've reached it," Barb proudly reported, yet her breathing had become more labored with every step.

"When I tell you to, turn to your left and walk out to the end of the platform, look out, and describe what you see. Do you understand?"

"I do," she replied, undaunted by her father's renewed but now pathetic threats. He no longer had any power over her. His voice sounded distant and frail. At the end of the platform she instantly caught a glimpse of a small brilliant ball of light entering her body from the right. She flinched at receiving it, and instinctively registered fear, but against all past knowledge and reactions she could then embrace its protective warmth. A thin, bright aura formed a cocoon around her like a second skin. She turned to face up the staircase and directed her reply to her father. *Listen, you asshole, I had to endure your alcoholic rages, beatings, sexual abuse, and torture but no longer. You trapped me. I was your daughter, but I'm done with you. No more. I'm in control from this point on. I am doing this for me, all of me. I choose recovery and health for me.* Barb bravely turned and took her first step down the staircase.

"From this point on, I have no daughter. I disown you forever," her father's voice declared in a last ditch effort to regain control.

Even under his intense threat of loss, Barb experienced a sensation of peace. The truth about her accomplishment came when the staircase went from darkness into light. She continued down to the twentieth step.

"I'm there, standing on the end of the platform," she proclaimed as another aspect of her history began to unfold in front of her. This time she was able to view the event without getting emotionally involved.

"Describe what you see?" Gooding interrupted.

"I see my living room with a man in it. My God, I don't believe it! It's my first husband sitting in that damn recliner with a beer in his hand. He's angry! Steven was always angry at everything."

"Who else do you see?"

"I don't see anyone else." Barb stated in confusion, her expression bewildered.

"Look around. Look around the house" Gooding said. "She has to be there. It's your image."

Barb went silent as her eyes darted back and forth under her eyelids searching for her missing self. Time lapsed as her frantic search continued.

"I found her. She's in the dining room rushing to put dinner on the table. Steven is getting angrier the longer she takes. She looks very worried. I'm scared for her."

"Don't take your eyes off her. Turn up your internal hearing and report what's being said," Gooding instructed.

Barb played the audio portion and repeated the words she was hearing in the image, "What the hell is taking you so long? You're such a stupid bitch that you can't even remember to cook my meals on time. You're a lousy wife."

Barb paused in fear as the man in the image began to berate the figure in the dining room. She had never confided to anyone how violent Steven became over the years. She had been too afraid because he would make her pay dearly if anyone found out about his abusive behavior. He threatened her all the time. The marriage had deteriorated from the minute the "lovely couple" had walked out of the church on their wedding day. Steven had transformed Barb from a human being into an "object" as soon as she said, "I do." She became his possession at that point.

Her thoughts drifted momentarily. At this point in her inner journey, she came to understand that the longer she kept her secrets hidden, the more inclined she was to protect them while becoming sicker and being further abused. She knew better, but in the past she just shut up and took it as her father had trained her to do.

She shook her head to disconnect from that thinking. She had a task to perform. *This has to stop once for all. I promise that from his point forward I will be loyal to me first, I swear.* She knew that her old patterns of loyalty must end here. Unable to dodge the spate of terror that followed, she stood and faced its onslaught. Her body locked up in fear. Her pulse raced, and she gasped for breath. Her face turned ashen, and her fingernails dug into the arms of the chair she sat in.

Gooding watched as Barb's affect made a sudden shift. Gooding instantly monitored her physical condition. She noted heart rate up, pulse up, and blood pressure up. Gooding assessed the situation quickly and diagnosed that Barb was getting hooked and about to be sucked into this image. Barb was about to relive the trauma. Gooding quickly intervened to let her know she had support. "Freeze the image. Take a breath. Just relax and describe what you see. I am here for you. You can do it. Don't let the image move. Hold it and don't judge, analyze, or interpret – just report!" Long pause. "That's it, you're doing it."

Barb knew what was occurring. It had happened before and was why she used anything and everything, to numb out. She wrestled for control, holding the image still while her body screamed in pain. Truly, before this program, this episode would have been enough to make her quit and terminate the incorporation process. Not this time. She had invested so much of herself in her program. She didn't fight it, didn't manipulate it, didn't cheat on it, didn't lie through it, didn't fake it, and didn't try to buy her way though it. Rather she challenged it and was trying to prove it didn't work. What she found was that the skills worked, and that was why she was attempting to complete the incorporation now. Barb forged on.

"Hang in there. You were right. We can't take it any longer. You can make it. I believe in you, and I'm with you all the way," came Annie's uncharacteristically soft and gentle voice, penetrating her mental struggle.

Barb couldn't respond. Her battle with fear was escalating, but she noted the support. Wave after wave attacked her small frame. This time she refused to back off or give in and she fought off every assault.

Gooding again noted tears being born in her eyes and carefully watched over her.

Barb was as vulnerable as a newborn babe at this stage of the process. Symbolically, she was indeed being born again. It would be the strength of her spirit and faith that would carry her home. Gooding's job was to keep her safe until she could guide her off the platform, back to going up the staircase, and back to the here and now.

On some level Barb was aware that Gooding was protecting her. She felt her presence on her left side. Her senses monitored someone else on her right side. Barb mentally looked around to see a shadowy figure approaching. It was Annie. For the first time she was able to clearly make out Annie's delicate face and discovered that Annie was smiling at her.

"I thought you had given up on me," Barb said.

"I did but I changed my mind. As the old saying goes, it's a lady's prerogative."

Back to back they returned to facing the attacks, and with reinforcement coming at the height of her pain threshold, the attacks ended.

"I always thought if you ignored the pain or kept in down, the problem would go away. I'm sorry I was wrong. Daddy was brutal to our body as well as our mind. I was there watching from a distance while you defeated him. When you battled with Daddy, I saw that he wasn't real, and he couldn't stop you. I'm no longer afraid of him. I have traveled through all the years with you. I'm sorry I abandoned you, but I'm back and here to stay. That is if you will have me," Annie said without allowing Barb to answer. Silence reigned as they still stood guard for yet another attack. *Of course, I've always needed you, and I can use the support. You forget that I created you to help me. I could never have survived him, Steven, or David without you.*

With a renewed passion for freedom she gathered her courage, her inner power, and went back to her task. Annie's silhouette returned to inside the image. Barb unfroze the image, reconnected and started to report again. Fragmented images of a knife flashed across her mental screen. "Steven is screaming at her. He is going into a violent rage. He always looked for an excuse. Oh, No! I have to get her out of there. Those eyes! He'll kill her this time. He's picking up the knife. God I can't look."

Gooding jumped in, "Don't take your eyes off her. Remember it happened it is not happening now."

"Don't abandon me again like you did that night." Annie pleaded from inside the image. "You left me trapped there to take the pain. You went to a place of no pain, but I couldn't escape.

You must look! I've had to carry our secrets all these years. You have to get through it this time so I can finally be free too. I know you perceived me as vile, dirty, and broken, just a nuisance, but I'm a part of you. Please rescue me. We can't continue to carry such massive secrets separately. We've paid our debts, so don't stop now." Barb's left hand increased in warmth as though Annie's hand was holding it.

I promise I won't abandon you ever again, Barb assured her.

She continued reporting to Gooding what she was observing. "It can't be true! Steven stabbed her with the knife! He actually pinned her hand to the table. Shit! She can't get away, she's trapped." Barb wanted to turn away, but she stood firm and sharpened in her resolve. "He's running around to the other side of the table. She can't get her hand loose. Wow! He is punching her in the face." She went back to giving an audio account of what Steven was saying. "Don't you ever defy me again, you slut." A long pause ensued while she witnessed the beating. "My meal is to be on time no matter what. You're nothing but a filthy whore. Bitch, you need to be taught a good lesson, one you'll never forget*.*" Steven laughed with glee. "You're father warned me about you, and he was right. You aren't worth shit!" Feeling the hurtful weight of his criticism, Barb reached deep within to reconnect with her spirituality. She had separated from her spirituality as a child, when she had begged God to please stop her father or let her die. No help had come then, so she was taking an enormous risk now. "She can't take any more. God, please don't let her die!" She begged as though she could change the outcome. "She'll never make it. The pain is incredible!" Even as she continued to witness the shocking events she sensed the therapist there at her side.

"I have been in total denial for a long time, but I didn't remember Steven being so brutal," she said, directing her comment to Gooding.

"It wasn't your fault. Continue if you want." Gooding replied to get her back on track.

"Please save her" Barb appealed again to her higher power. She took a quick breath and described the scene. "He's behind her. Steven is touching her private parts while she is pinned to the table and bleeding. She is getting weak. He's sick! It's too much to watch."

"Do you want to save her?" Said Gooding cutting through her emotional intensity. Puzzlement filled Barb's brain. For a fraction of a second, she considered the possibility and the consequences, good and bad, she would have to risk.

"Do you want to rescue her?" Gooding said with even more passion.

"Yes, yes I do!"

"Then freeze the image."

"I don't know if I can. I'm afraid."

"Freeze the image." Gooding demanded urgently. "You have the power. You didn't work this hard to give up now; you didn't come all this way to quit. Once you freeze it you can safely enter the image and save her. Let me know as soon as you have it frozen." Gooding delivered more instructions, "Don't hesitate, don't think; run off the platform into the image. Stand in between 'self' and Steven. He can't hurt or stop you. Let me know when it's so. Tell me when you are there."

Mounting all her resources, Barb gave one last mental push and the image paused. "It's frozen. I have to get her out of there!" She blurted with great relief.

Barb skillfully worked her way through the image and stood face to face with Steven in the frozen frame. Fear burgeoned, but she completed the task. "Okay, I'm there."

"Would you like to do or say anything to Steven?" Gooding had felt Barb strongly needed revenge.

"I do."

"If you have a need, look down to your right. You'll see a two-by-four on the floor. Do you see it?"

"I do."

"Pick it up and use it to do whatever you want to Steven, or use it for protection. Say whatever you have to say to him. Let me know as soon as you're done. Do you understand?"

"Yes."

Gooding watched as Barb's temporary helplessness turned to strength and monitored her heart rate and breathing. She wanted to be ready in case Barb needed intervention.

Barb hesitated but a second before going into action. In her mind she grabbed him by the throat and threw him across the room. She walked over to him and beat him with the board, venting all her pent-up rage. "I won't let you do that to her any more!" she shouted. "I'm done," she announced to Gooding.

"Then drop the board and turn so you are facing 'self'. Remove the knife from her hand, pick her up in your arms, and bring her back to the platform. He can't stop you or hurt you. Tell me when you have her back." Barb did what she asked.

"I have her in my arms and we are back," she stated with personal authority.

"Both of you are safe on the platform, and the image is fading. He can't hurt you ever again," she said to self.

More instructions from Gooding "Now hold her lovingly, look into her eyes, and repeat after me."

Barb nodded okay and spoke right after her. "I love you; I'm sorry I left you. I was so overwhelmed that I had to go. The pain and fear were so intense that I thought I was going to die. I had to escape the only way I knew how. I came back today to rescue you because I can no longer live without you or in pieces. I see that you weren't to blame for what happened. I want you to come and live inside with me so that we can be whole, happy, and healthy, safe and protected, complete, and confident. For the first time in our lives we can live free from all past pain and hurt. If you'll do that, I promise never ever to shame, blame, reject, discount, dismiss, or abandon you. I truly love you." The relaxation of her body gave witness to her level of commitment.

"Now, with the adult 'self' in your arms, turn 180 degrees, climb back up the stairs, turn right, and go on up. Run as fast as you want all the way back to the platform where you left the little girl. Let me know when you get there."

"I'm there," Barb said after minutes of silence.

"All right, turn around, and you'll see me behind you." Gooding paused.

"Do you see me?"

"I do."

"Hand me the adult 'self' you have in your arms."

"Okay."

"Now turn around and pick up the little girl sitting on the platform. Good. Return to the staircase, holding her tightly. Turn right and go as fast as you want up to the top platform you built when we began. Let me know when you're there and I'll follow with your adult self in my arms. Nothing can stop you. Let me know when you reach the top." Gooding witnessed an increase in her breathing rate as though she were making a physical effort.

"We're there!" a breathless Barb proclaimed.

"Turn around again and face me. I'm now handing you your adult self. You can hold both of them in your arms, lovingly and safely. Let me know when you have them."

"I do."

"Now turn 180 degrees and look toward the other end of the platform. You'll see a line of three square concrete patio blocks floating just off the end. Do you see them?"

"I do."

"Now with the child and the woman in your arms, walk out to the farthest block. It will support and protect all three of you; acknowledge as soon as you are there."

"We're there," Barb said in joyful voice.

Gooding continued her instructions. "The two patio blocks, the platform, and the staircase will disappear in what seems to be water. You're now cut off from all past hurt, pain, rejection, and abandonment. But you need to focus your attention on the two in your arms and repeat after me: I love you both. I'm so sorry, but I thought that I was about to die. I admit that I abandoned you. I'm here to rescue you because I can no longer live in fragmented pieces. I now know that neither you nor I are to blame for what happened. I want you both to come and live with me." Barb repeated it all.

Her capability and enthusiasm were now congruent with her words. She grew stronger with every instruction she followed.

"Using your arms, pull them in towards your chest," Gooding said. Barb followed through. She felt the two self figures being symbolically absorbed into the gaping hole that had been present in her chest for as long as she could remember. It was like fitting in the right piece of a puzzle to finish the picture. She sensed entry of her soul and spirit. The warmth of wholeness encompassed her. She had always thought she was missing part of herself, and that feeling of separateness had just vanished. Wondrous, creative thoughts and emotions traveled along her mental circuits, replacing the terror and negativism. For the first time since her infancy, Barb became aware that her head was unified with her body.

"As you stand there alone on that patio block, look deep into the dark in front of you," said Gooding. "You'll see the dot you put behind your forehead when you started the procedure. Tell me as soon as you see it."

"I see it," Barb answered.

At your leisure, walk off the patio block toward that dot. As you move closer to it you'll be returning safely to the present, bringing your wholeness with you. As soon as you are back to the here and now, I want you to open your eyes."

Barb could hardly contain her excitement as she rushed toward the dot. United with it she became conscious of how heavy her eyelids felt from being closed so long. Taking a gulp of fresh air, she began to open them. She sat motionless in the chair, attempting to attune her senses to reality. For a second she feared her sense of peacefulness would vanish if she moved. "I can look back at what happened without pain or fear. I checked. I understand how I have kept that part of me separated from the light," she said.

She continued to bask in the wholesome glow for a few more minutes. Gooding offered some insight into the pledges she had made to herself and some after effects that she might expect. She congratulated Barb on an incredible accomplishment. "You're free to fly. Your life is what you make of it from this point on," she said as she opened the office door for her.

Barb returned to the unit with a sense of completeness and happiness that pulsated through her entire being. She instinctively knew her dreadful journey was over, but that another had just begun. While walking along the hall, Barb looked around to see if she was alone. Her eyes sparkled with self-affirmation as a childish smile spread across her face. "This one is for you Annie," Barb said as she skipped the rest of the way to her room.

Part 2

Instruction

Chapter 5

"What Do I Need to Change?"

The first thing that needs to change is attitude.

- recovery is possible.
- there is a different way to recover.
- success is possible.

1. How can anyone challenge what isn't understood?

Prior to the onset of intrusive posttraumatic stress symptoms, (exaggerated responses, detachment, anger, depression, flashbacks, loss of interest in life, mood swings, hypervigilance, time loss, intrusive thoughts, recurrent dreams, avoidance, inappropriate feelings) the person had functioned satisfactorily. But once the intrusive period begins, she doesn't understand why or where the fragmented pieces of information come from. Mind and body cannot validate them, so the response is to deny, ignore, withdraw, and isolate from others and life.

2. How can anyone challenge what isn't known?

The suddenly invading material can't be explained by examining a person's environment or known past history. She has thoughts like "What bad things have I done to deserve this?" or "I've gone crazy!" or "Am I making all this up?" Without some type of validation she is left with heavy doubt and pondering whether or not one or more of those thoughts about herself might be true.

3. How can anyone challenge what isn't seen?

The only evidence of the victim's tortuous experiences are the images locked inside her mind. PTSD is not like a broken bone that can be seen in an x-ray or a blocked colon that can be surgically opened to reveal an obstruction. Since other people can't see the reasons for her distress, or corroborate her experiences, she often denies what she is seeing in her own head. "After all, if no one else can see the reasons for my distress perhaps there aren't any."

As you continue reading, please think about the three questions just presented. Ponder what you might think about yourself if you were having persistent negative thoughts, emotions, and behaviors, and had no perceivable explanation for their cause.

Natural disasters and man's inhumanity to man have been going on since the dawn of time. Now, because of technology, the media gives us access to many catastrophic events as they are happening or mere seconds after they occur. We have witnessed actual firefights in wars, the horror of the World Trade Center collapse, and the tragedy of families whose children have been abducted and murdered. Even the ravages of past storms, earthquakes, and volcanic eruptions are continuously broadcast into the supposed safety of our living rooms.

Because of this media invasion there are people in our society walking around suffering secondary PTSD that don't even know they have it. They don't recognize their symptoms or understand why they might be hurting. Also affected are first hand victims of emotional, physical, verbal, and sexual trauma, as their symptoms are triggered and exacerbated.

"Is there any hope?" is the most common question asked of me. At the time of their first traumatic experience, survivors hoped with all their heart to be rescued or allowed to die, but no one or nothing saved them. The lesson learned was that hope was out of their reach; for some reason they didn't deserve to be saved. From that point on they felt condemned to a life of torment for being broken, crippled, defective, dirty, bad, damaged, or incomplete. Not wanting people to know, they lock themselves behind a veil of secrecy that they keep in place at all costs. Even though what was done horrified them, they became bonded to the source of their pain. This devotion to the perpetrator soon turned to deep loyalty, causing them to take the anger and disgust engendered by the experience and turn it in on themselves.

Let's examine the common definition of hope: "a desire with expectation of fulfillment." Hope flares in the midst of trauma. People hope for release from the pain and terror as the incidents occur, they hope they'll wake up and discover it was all a nightmare, and later when their symptoms became too much to bear they hope for a cure. None occurs, and the pain continues and the invasive symptoms never seem to let up. Eventually, after endless waiting, longing, and broken expectations, hope is abandoned. The good things they had hoped for seem to happen only to others.

The ensuing hopelessness causes them to analyze, interpret, and judge their thoughts, actions, and feelings. They believe they are what others have taught them to be. They feel that everyone else is more correct than they. Self-doubting becomes a way of life. They live a pseudo existence, half in and half out of reality that blocks their ability to live in the present. They rely on others (abuser, family members, peers, teachers, coaches, spouses, relationships, and bosses) to define who they are and how they should think, act, and feel.

Due to a perceived defectiveness, all their mental and physical power goes into being a "perfect person." They develop incorrect assumptions that say "If I were perfect the hurting would stop." "If I were perfect I'd be loved." Of course they never attain that level of perfection, so again they fail, and their dislike for self grows. Consequently their self is sentenced to roam the earth in a state of numbness.

Another aspect of hope occurs on a spiritual level. Those trapped in trauma will at some point turn their eyes to the heavens and beg for spiritual intervention. They ask that the pain and hurt be stopped, or that they be taken up into Heaven. Nothing happens. No one materializes to combat the source of trauma, and they remain alive. Because rescue didn't happen they decide that the God of their understanding isn't real, or they think their requests were denied because they themselves were worthless, damaged, defective or not good enough to save. They believe that their God or "higher power" had rejected and abandoned them. Their relationship with their God suffers greatly and they begin to discard their spiritual beliefs. Their new belief that develops is "What can't be seen or touched isn't real."

As a result of spiritual conflict, loneliness develops within them. Their spiritual selves are overshadowed by a life of seeking definition, fulfillment, love, and validation from other people. They perceive that whatever might stop their suffering has to come from someone else. They no longer think that anything good can emerge from within. They rationalize that validation of self is only achieved through being loved by someone, materialism, status, or belonging to a group. They reach outside self looking for that right person, job, technique, drug, or object that will banish their loneliness, fill their emptiness, and give them piece of mind. Failed effort after failed effort, they grow disillusioned over the years. Fear becomes their reality because nothing stops the pain.

As if the preceeding symptoms weren't enough, they also face a constant barrage of internal negative messages and thoughts that seem to control their thinking, feelings, and behaviors in their relationships to self and the world. Posttraumatic stress symptoms appear: flashbacks, body memories, intrusive thoughts, inappropriate behavior, nightmares, and body pains. Their lives seem meaningless, devoid of emotion, and incomplete. They recognize a loss of control of self and their daily lives. From that point on thoughts, feelings, and behaviors adhere to a set of guidelines, commands, messages and values that stream through their own minds. They truly believe there is no hope for self.

A feeling of loss grows deep within, accompanied by the knowledge that their experience of self is different from that of other people. A sensation of emptiness begins to surface in their chest. They focus more and more on that difference, obscuring the ability to see their own uniqueness. As a result they sink progressively into feelings of helplessness, hopelessness, loneliness, fear, and depression. Self becomes isolated in an interior prison.

So is there hope?

On one hand the answer is simple, a positive *yes*. There is hope for a life, a future; and yes, there is a way back.

The first step in getting better is to knock down the distorted perceptions that people who go through trauma are weak and defective. I know that survivors are certainly neither. Those who come through serious trauma do so because in truth they are strong, intelligent, powerful, and creative. Anyone who hasn't experienced profound trauma can't understand the resources it takes to endure such an overwhelming event. It requires a massive amount of internal power and cooperation between mind, body, and spirit to complete the survival process. The ability to survive is a gift, an incredible miracle. The mechanism that assists in that process is given to people before they're born. If someone comes face-to-face with an intensely traumatic event and struggles to live through it, the gift is activated allowing that person symbolically to separate the head (cognition) from the body (emotions/pain). The separation permits the denial of the event and the pain through a symbolic escape unseen by the hurting source. But alas, since that gift can't be demonstrated on demand or scientifically duplicated in a laboratory, it isn't recognized by our society, but is seen as a pathological defect.

Surviving trauma takes the ability to instinctively and unconsciously channel one's power, strength, intelligence, and creativity into saving their core, the essence of one's self. The gift described above allows the core to be hidden for protection somewhere within the body so it can't be captured by the invading traumatizing source. Self becomes unavailable. After the passage of time a traumatized person doesn't remember the location of the hidden core or its importance.

On the other hand there is much debate about hope and its involvement in recovery. Without hope there is no future. Unfortunately, hope isn't the only ingredient of successful therapy, nor is it scientific. So, does it exist? Yes, there is hope for recovery.

Hope is a creation of self born of the imagination, but hope can't come to fruition alone. It needs help through action and that is hard work. For recovery the sufferer needs to endure no matter what it takes. There will be struggle in both the action and the follow through, but if the goal is worthwhile, the struggle is worthwhile. A key to surviving the struggle is faith.

Faith

Real growth and recovery can only be achieved in an atmosphere of faith. Life is more than things and events you can see, smell, or touch. Living requires a great deal of faith, the ability to believe in something that's not visible in the moment. Faith can be seen in the act of following through on something when there's no logical proof or material evidence promising success. When the steps toward recovery require a person to walk down frighteningly unfamiliar pathways, it's only faith in the experience of others or faith in the process that keeps one from running.

Faith needs to be maintained on a daily basis. It's nurtured through group support; one on one sharing, prayer, internal communication, deep personal reflection, or meditation and reading material. Faith can help you deal with things that you've never been able to cope with before. It's the thing that allows you to believe in the truth, value and worthiness of your inner self.

The Three Dirtiest Words in the World

The journey of recovery has many unknown barriers, among which are what we refer to as "the three dirtiest words in the world:" **decisions, responsibilities,** and **consequences.**

Rule number one is "Don't make any decisions." The victim takes rigid control of her thoughts. She no longer trusts her inner self. She won't make any *decisions* that conflict with the covert rules which formed from her trauma experience.

Rule number two is if the victim doesn't make the decision which governs her action, then she incurs no *responsibility* for the outcome of that action.

Rule number three is that all negative *consequences* are deserved.

Rule number four supports the first three: Never, ever make friends with self as that will lead to violations of the other three.

Overcoming the distorted mindset around these three words requires their redefinition and understanding them in a better way.

Decision is defined as: a) the act or process of deciding or b) a determination arrived at after consideration. It means making a choice or a conclusion.

The nature of a traumatic experience makes the person feel as if a bad decision may have caused the event (took the wrong bus, wore the wrong clothes, said the wrong thing). Trauma takes away her decision-making ability. From that point on she questions, doubts, judges and distrusts any decision for fear that being wrong again will bring further pain. The unconscious lesson learned from trauma is that safety, acceptance and love come only from letting other people govern her decisions. She now views her own thinking as a problem.

Prior to entering recovery the victim must decide between living with the symptoms of PTSD or recovering. Both cannot be done at the same time. I believe that the person has to grab for personal authority in order to recover from the effects of trauma. It is a person's right to choose how they think, act or feel. A person survives horrible events by not yielding to an overwhelming force, but creating alternate paths to preservation. Whether the person consciously remembers it or not, she made a decision to live.

To become active in recovery, the person needs to make a strong decision to recover. The person must be willing to commit to that decision no matter what. No matter how tempting or beneficial looking some other offer might be, the decision must be kept. The decision for recovery is manifest in the act of taking back control of thoughts, emotions, and behavior that were usurped by the trauma. Doing what was deemed unwise.

Once that decision has been made, the person must readjust attitudes and perception of what recovery does or does not mean. The person needs to give up the unreachable goal of some imagined state of perfection and begin to see life for what it really is: a unique challenge full of unpredictable circumstances, events, and feelings that are sometimes pleasant and sometimes painful. But half of the enjoyment of living is being involved. Making ones own decisions doesn't guarantee the outcome will always be desirable, but every person should have the right to decide for self.

Responsibility is defined as: (1) the act of being answerable for actions or decisions; (2) the ability to respond appropriately. I define it as being true to one's word to self, and the natural outcome of making a decision. It doesn't mean accepting someone else's word: "you are a failure". It doesn't mean meeting someone else's expectations: "why aren't you like your older sister". Nor does it mean being accountable to someone else's values that are forced upon you: "You are worthless." I believe that no one can be held responsible for an act, emotion, or thought that wasn't agreed to or accepted or that was forced upon them. Be true to promises made by self.

The last dirty word of our trio is *consequences,* defined as (1) something produced by a cause or following from a given set of conditions and (2) the result or effect. Rule number three in this section says that all negative results and their consequences are deserved. Trauma results are never positive. Even though a person is the victim, they take negative consequences for everyone else's decisions. The skill of accepting positive consequences is never learned. Yet to grow and become mature the person must learn to accept the consequences of their own actions, whether the consequence is accepting compliments for succeeding at a task or criticisms for not completing a task. Consequences stem from following through or not following through on a decision. The result or effect of any act may be good, bad or indifferent.

Decisions are what make people human. All decisions influence behaviors, thoughts and feelings. I truly believe that all of us have the right to make our own decisions without fear, force, or threat.

Incongruent Messages

It's important to understand what is meant by incongruent messages in order to move forward. They are dissimilar, contradictory, or unrelated statements that register in the brain during a traumatic experience such as rape. In the midst of a repugnant, physically painful, and emotionally overwhelming event, the victim is told, "This will feel so good you'll like it. If you love me you'll let me do this" when in fact the body is in terrible pain. Messages like "You're feeling good makes me know how special you are to me" when the one speaking of love is the abuser. The victim feels dirty and showers all the time but never feels clean. Though she's told by others she's pretty, she sees herself as broken, damaged and defective even when the mirror says differently.

There are other incongruent messages: "What you think and feel is wrong; I am always right. You'll never amount to anything and no one will ever want you. You're nothing without me. Promise you will never tell because you know you wanted it. You are no better than me because you liked it." Such statements foster damaging patterns of self-hate years after the initial event. Incongruent messages create a conflict between internal truth and the forced pseudo reality of the victim's life.

Trauma entraps the body, making it feel empty and foreign. After emerging from trauma, the brain is inundated with a continuous barrage of messages. The victim levels endless shame, blame and guilt onto self. The victim begins trusting only information and validation from outside of self. She searchs for ways to fix or disown the incongruent messages and to make self more acceptable to others; but finds no answer. The end result is a self which is no longer listened to or trusted.

The victim grows up listening to incongruent messages. So everyday life is simple; 'since I can't trust myself I'll just do as I'm told.' Deep inside, her truth is yearning for a normal life, hoping somehow to be magically transformed into being congruent with the rest of the world, no longer out of step.

Foundation for personal reconstruction

Trauma created a foundation of thoughts, perceptions, truths, and values upon which self developed. Think of it this way: A person lives in a house built to someone else's specifications. It doesn't fit her. It has short walls and low ceilings; it's filled with values, beliefs, and perceptions that are not the survivor's. The windows are lenses that filter the view of the world and distort all information. The doors are sealed shut. There are no exits. Everything inside is unfamiliar, scary, and dark. Trapped forever?

No. There is a way out – she needs to build a house to her own self specifications. Knowledge was controlled and normalcy distorted. Truth was ignored and lies were used as the tool of control. So education is the foundation on which to build anew. If she decides to leave the familiar, education offers fertile ground on which to create a comfortable, safe, and growth-oriented environment. As anyone who has built a house knows, the experience is not without anxiety that produces fears and doubts. Yet once built, the house fits the owner's needs. Of course building the shell is not the end of the job; but the beginning. With the outer structure completed, her creative energy needs to focus on interior decorating and daily management.

The experience of early trauma robs the victim of all that should have been learned during her formative years. It isolates her in a world of dark secrets, fear, and hurt. After losing developmental years through trauma, how does she reinvent self? She should design the real self she wants, the person she would like to be. The process of creating anew I call designing a self-concept. It's just like blue printing and building a house. Developing a self-concept is not easy; it takes good planning, patience, constant vigilance, and hard work. From design through implementation, periods of discouragement and doubt will interrupt the process. She must deal with them openly, consciously exploring new behavior patterns, habits, and attitudes. If parts of the self-concept don't work or don't fit, then she ought to explore new information, absorb it and use it to form a mindset of self-empowerment, self-values, and self-validation. Studies show that the more information a person has about a task, the easier it is to perform. Increased learning correlates directly with reducing the anxiety and fear related to any task, thus increasing the possibility of success.

Education is the light that helps the victim out of the darkness and to see self as normal. Normal in that anyone put through the same type of trauma, at the same age would have the same symptoms. Learning helps her to understand that self reacted normally to an abnormal circumstance. She can begin to understand her emotions and thoughts not as crazy but as being responsive to a distorted situation.

Education is the act of gathering information that leads to learning, learning to knowledge, and knowledge to wisdom. Wisdom empowers.

Chapter 6

The Unfolding Self

The miracle that is a human being is seen in the complexity of all the interrelated systems that go into making up the whole. In past research the emphasis on trauma has focused on dissecting a victim into malfunctioning systems or specific symptoms rather than on understanding the person as a whole system. Everyone is unique. No two people react to the same stimulus in exactly the same way, so each must be studied as a complete entity if their strengths, powers, and weaknesses are to be understood. After all, it is as a unit that the human system interacts with its environment while relating to its own internal reality and spiritual world.

Accomplishing a balance between internal reality and external reality is a monumental task in our fast-paced, technological world. Our society de-emphasizes individuality in favor of sameness. There are too many expectations that decrease the time available for self. They can keep a person constantly focused on external validation and staying in balance. Yet it is internal balance and validation that fosters a sense of wholeness. When a person's system is out of balance and self is invalidated, the individual experiences hopelessness, depression, and internal chaos.

A common factor found in trauma survivors is the failure to understand what happened. If they were successful at the act of survival and achieved a dissociative state in order to escape the overwhelming trauma, they don't remember it. As a result of the traumatic event the victim's development and maturity are stunted at that age, and they lose a sense of self. They carry a growing feeling of emptiness and worthlessness. Then out of the blue in adulthood, their ability to function in the world crumbles, and chaos intrudes upon their thoughts and emotions. The victim feels as though they've entered an area of total blackness. They withdraw and become uncomfortable around others. They trust no one from then on, especially self. They experience feeling broken, incomplete, damaged, and defective, with a growing sensation of emptiness like there's a hole in the middle of their chests. It feels as if a part of them is missing.

At some point after the initial trauma, a victim's symptoms become intrusive. They start viewing flashbacks of the trauma. Hence the word post in PTSD, which means the symptoms may not appear for weeks, months, or years after the original event. Inexplicable pain, and disturbing images disrupt their days and haunt their nights. The loss of memory of childhood events makes the person feel as if the surfacing fragmented images are generated from an unknown source with no link to any identifiable memory. Accompanying the images come intense levels of emotional pain and physical discomfort. Frightened and confused, the person really believes that craziness has taken over. The more the person can't explain or relate to the fragmented images and the emotional suffering, the more they attempt to deny or "numb out" the pain that is happening. By ignoring it that way the victim actually increases the intensity of the memories. Inability to predict or control these occurrences, increase the person's levels of fear, anxiety, and feelings of being out of control, that then become the dominant focus in their life. They anxiously monitor both inner thoughts and the external environment while waiting for the next invasion of fragmented images. Having no control over these episodes that feel so emotionally and physically real, they promise self never to let anyone know what's going on inside. They live in secrets, unable to find any rational explanation for the incongruent experiences within, learning not to trust any of self's thoughts, judgments, or feelings. They judge as weakness or defectiveness their inability to explain their internal experiences and translate them into feelings. Therefore they disown large pieces of themselves and simply give up. Considering self as toxic the suffering person withdraws into the darkness of silence and self-isolation to avoid contaminating other people, particularly loved ones.

The sufferer spends their time trying to stop the pain of the past from invading the present. They believe no future is deserved until the past is resolved. They reason that no one would ever want someone who is defective and damaged, so they become stuck, isolated, not experiencing the present and not planning for the future. Trying to defend self consumes their energy. The victim reasons that if self does nothing (withdraws, hides, and isolates), then self can't be accused of doing anything wrong (stupid, inadequate or imperfect). Although the person doesn't understand what's happening, self becomes painfully aware that life exists without light. Total loneliness and darkness set in.

At that point the person feels controlled by others and is subject to forces outside of self. They automatically act and feel other people's perceptions, values, and expectations. Living that way erodes their self-confidence, self-worth, self-image, and self-esteem. The person has no concept of who self is and can only perform according to what has been witnessed and taught. The external world demands demonstrations of loyalty in every aspect of life (family, country, employment, school, social organizations). All the person feels inside is emptiness, pain, abandonment, and loss along with fear and anxiety that increase daily. All trust is gone.

From this point forward I will be presenting my theory and principles about the structure that the survival process may take inside a victim. The strength, creativity, intelligence and power a person uses in order to restructure and reorganize internal systems. This process allows a person to escape the overwhelming emotional pain of a trauma. Escape is necessary because the person has no defenses. I believe that the ability to survive is a creative, internal process, not visible to the outside world, and that survival occurs on a purely symbolic basis.

The following is very important for developing a basic philosophy of survival. *I believe that my clients are victims who used their inherent strengths, creativity, intelligence and power to survive.* Survival is not the result of illness or defectiveness, but of the human characteristics of strength, creativity, intelligence and power. To recover a person must believe those characteristics are worth saving and use them to recover. The first step is to learn how the survival process works and how wondrous it is. The survival reaction is a normal response to an abnormal situation. What follows is the theory I teach to the survivors I work with.

Wholeness of Self

I have developed a theory and principles to describe the survival process which I term the process of *symbolic unfolding*. The following sections describe that process as it relates to the internal reaction of a victim to a single incident or repetitive episodes of trauma.

Let me start with defining the word *whole* as it fits my theory. Whole is the state of having all the proper parts or components or in one unit. It is the state of being in balance. Wholeness is the act of all human systems being in harmony, but it doesn't require any kind of perfection.

The first principle is that human beings are born whole, in a state where all systems are in balance. Wholeness is represented as a circle (Diagram 1). Everyone has a boundary (skin) and a core. A protective boundary surrounds the core, forming a safe area for growth. The core harbors a blueprint of the basic characteristics that make up a person's essence, spirituality, uniqueness, identity, esteem, imaginativeness, genuineness, and depth. The blueprint contains the basic elements of that person's makeup (RNA and DNA). My principle states that the core must be protected at all costs. If the core is ever damaged or symbolically captured, self cannot be what it is meant to be.

I define *trauma* as (1) any life event that causes mental, emotional or physical unbalance with lasting emotional, physical, spiritual or psychic effects (2) any event that causes self to feel invaded emotionally, physically or spiritually. Symbolically it is the fear of possible capture of the core that motivates the unfolding process. Were the core to be captured, the person couldn't return to a state of balance.

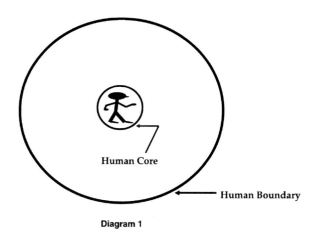

THE WHOLE SELF
Symbolic Configuration of a Human in Balance at Birth

Diagram 1

An example of the core's significance is to liken it to a motherboard in a computer that determines how all the parts interact and run as a whole machine. If the motherboard is damaged or removed, the computer can't function as it was meant to. The human core works in much the same way, coordinating the systems and determining the characteristics of the whole.

Movement of Self

If a person develops after birth without experiencing trauma, either primary (when it happens to the individual) or secondary (when it is witnessed by the individual), their developmental process will progress towards health. The first seven years of life constitute the most important period of growth and personality formation. If those years are trauma-free, a solid foundation forms on which personality can grow.

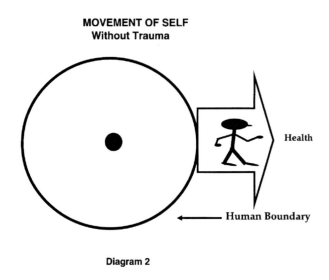

Diagram 2

In the normal developmental process there are three periods:

0-7 – Creating the Foundation for personality

7-19 – Building Personality on that foundation

19+ - Practice and fine tuning personality

Conversely if an individual experiences trauma that is overwhelmingly emotionally painful and there is no physical escape possible, internal escape in the form of imagining that the event is not occurring or mental relocation takes place. It distances and protects self from the horror of reality (Diagram 3). When the fear escalates to an unsupportable level along with a feeling of being trapped, it becomes vital to preserve the core from capture at all costs. Physical, mental, and spiritual systems unite to hide the core and insure its survival.

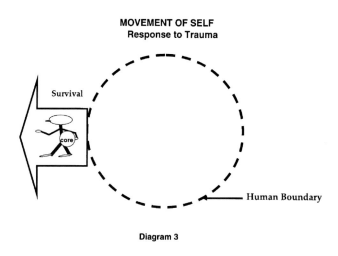

Diagram 3

The core is lovingly hidden within a maze of symbolic compartments that isolate it from the real world and guard against its capture. The process of hiding the core is what I term *unfolding the whole self into parts*. This act shields the core from damage it would suffer by exposure to pain or to further trauma. To protect the core's location the hiding is done without the person's knowledge. Unfortunately, the experience is later perceived by the person as a devastating loss of self.

To envision the symbolic unfolding think of the head (mental system) assisted by the imagination disconnecting from the body (physical system) (Diagram 4). It's much like an escape pod separating from the mother shuttle. The body may be frozen in terror, bound and gagged, trapped under a building, or hurled through a windshield, but the mind never stops wanting to protect self. Regardless of age, as long as the mind is active and the decision to live is made, the whole will seek survival.

Internal Mental Escape in Response to Trauma (Dissociation)

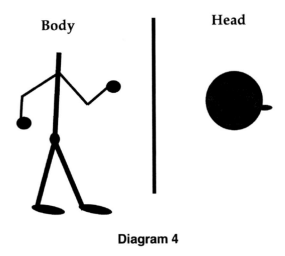

Diagram 4

I strongly believe that the availability of the unfolding process is a gift present at birth. Regrettably, sometimes it's insufficient and the victim doesn't survive. The miracle is that the majority of the traumatized do complete the survival process.

Elements of Movement

Movement on the continuum (Diagram 5) is the act of passing through a series of unfolding stages to distance self from the pain of reality. The distance someone moves up the continuum is based on the six elements, individually or collectively.

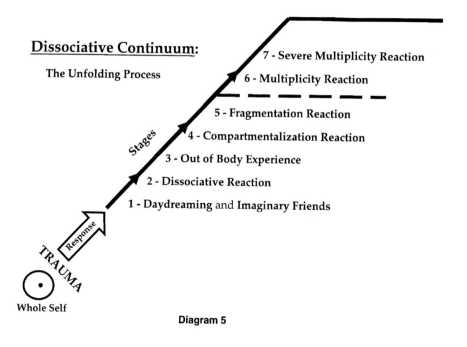

Diagram 5

Element 1. **Degree of Sensitivity**

Everyone is born with different sensitivity levels and varying degrees of toleration. What might be traumatic to one person could be exciting to another. Sensitivity seems to be the main element that determines response and reaction to any event. It determines the perception of whether the associated emotion will be interpreted as positive, negative, or indifferent.

Element 2. **Age at Time of First Trauma**

The human brain is most impressionable between birth and seven years of age when the personality is in flux and building a foundation. During that period of rapid growth the personality is at its most vulnerable. The brain takes in and stores more information then than in any other developmental stage.

The younger the person is at the time of the trauma, fewer are the mental filters to process incoming data (all thoughts, feelings, sensations and behaviors). All information is therefore accepted as truth. Formation of mental filters happens out of experience with reality, distorted or not. Experiences are judged at their conclusion and stored. That stored information becomes a foundation for the next experience to be filtered through. Filters determine future reactions to life events.

Stored information distorted or not, shapes a person's attitudes behaviors doubts, fears, feelings, hopes, knowledge, needs, prejudices, thoughts, views and wants. How that person will function is based on the information, and it determines how creative movement up the continuum will be.

Element 3. **Repetitiveness**

Repetitiveness refers specifically to the amount of trauma and how often traumatic acts are experienced. Their frequency determines the number of stages a person must move along the continuum to distance self from frequent, overwhelming emotional pain and loss. With each incident resistance decreases, increasing movement up the continuum.

Element 4. **Severity**

Severity is in the eyes of the beholder, in this case the one being hurt. Severity refers to the intensity and degree of violence perceived. It influences the response, and increases the necessity to hide further up the continuun.

Element 5. **Amount of pain**

Pain relates directly to the individuals perception of how much can be tolerated. There are different types of pain – mental, emotional, spiritual, and physical. Everyone has a different pain threshold for each type. There is a threshold at which the whole will begin to break down and be vulnerable from then on. How much pain will be tolerated is based on that ultimate threshold.

Element 6. **Degree of Need**

This element refers to the intensity of a specific need. Each person has different needs. Examples of a few different types are: the need to attach, to belong, to be recognized; the need for control and for power. It is the degree that determines how much focus, drive, and importance is given to some needs over others.

The Miraculous Unfolding of Self

The foregoing elements are the motivators for movement on the continuum, i.e. the degree of unfolding needed to survive. The unfolding process is truly astonishing. From a symbolic viewpoint, unfolding is a gift from God or higher power, an act of self-protection, and self-love. It's an imaginative response to a threat against the whole, an innate internal reaction. Unfolding is a way to creatively combat the negative effects of various kinds of trauma. It is activated only when all defenses are overwhelmed and no other avenue of escape is possible. It is activated when a child is presented with only two options, death or creative rescue. Is the child to accept reality and pain, be overwhelmed, possibly die, or does it escape through the imagination to attain survival? More often than not, people make the decision to live and create alternative defenses to that end. Creating alternative defenses is the unfolding of self. The process involves breaking down the whole human system into parts. It can be likened to a nation that separates into many little countries, each of which gradually develops more independence and less collectivity.

This process is not visible to the outside world and happens on a symbolic level with everyone's choice of symbols being unique. The unfolding process itself is a very personal and spiritual experience. I believe each person is a culture unto them self. How they record an event, judge and then respond is based on their age at the time of the first trauma, race, region raised in, education, values (family, religion, and country), environment, economic level, and social status. Those are also components of a culture in the general sense.

Summary

A. Progression from one stage to the next depends on the degree of the six elements of movement - sensitivity, extent of need, age at first trauma, frequency, severity, and increase in intensity.

B. The unfolding of self can happen at any age in reaction to trauma that is perceived as an overwhelming sense of loss, feelings of terror, and fear of dying. At the point where all control is lost, all defenses fail, or the body is trapped with no avenue of physical escape, the head symbolically separates from the body. It is an instinctive occurrence designed to preserve the whole, allowing thought to continue while emotional pain is avoided. An intense internal conflict evolves between the head and the body. The self initially unfolds into two parts, neither of which can accept or forgive the other. After all, the mind thinks the body failed to stop the trauma; the body feels that the head has rejected and abandoned it. Mind and body disown each other. The body subsequently becomes the head's target for self-punishment, criticism, blame, and hatred.

C. A young child reacts to trauma instinctively, feeling scared, helpless, defenseless, empty, hopeless, terrorized, out of control, and alone. The child did the best it could in the circumstances and should be celebrated for it. It isn't fair for a grown-up using adult criteria to judge, analyze, or interpret the unfolding reaction of self done by a trapped child many years ago.

D. Trauma must be viewed according to the child's age at its onset. When the child perceives that pain comes from the outside it will logically turn inward for protection. Finding no way out, it connects with its spirituality for help ("Please God, I don't want to die"). In response to the plea a collective union forms between the imagination, mind, body, and spirit to facilitate survival (the unfolding). Children think in symbols. When symbolic thought becomes part of the protective process, it is very personal and is only viewed accurately through the age appropriate eyes of the child during the trauma.

E. Because the unfolding process is symbolic, it cannot be fully understood on a literal basis. Symbolic thinking creates a polarization of the issues into extremes: light or dark, safety or vulnerability, life or death, joy or pain, good or bad, love or hate, silence or rage.

F. The unique unfolding or complicated defensive process involves the interaction of every internal system a person is graced with. Therefore, understanding the unfolding process may offer some clue to helping the person toward recovery. Recovering may come through figuring out the person's symbolism and creating a structure that uses the same symbols as tools to reverse the process. The way to recovery may be found in the person's imagination.

G. All the information taken in during a trauma results in the construction of a series of distorted mental filters that color perception of reality and relationship with self. Positive, negative, or neutral perceptions are formed by what the victim absorbed at the time of the trauma and affects every area of that person's development, choices, feelings, actions, and interactions.

H. A victim of trauma mentally escapes into the head by performing the act of dissociating, and the body is left trapped in the event to experience the physical horrors. The protective reaction of dissociating is the ability to make what is real into something unreal. Without this ability the person would be overwhelmed and die.

I. The extent of unfolding depends on the elements of movement discussed earlier. A complete unfolding of self (Multiplicity Reaction {DID}) only occurs within a child under the age of seven who experiences high levels of all of the elements of movement. Older children and adults who encounter the same levels of trauma and losses can't unfold as far because the personalities, characteristics, and defenses have already developed.

The Unfolding of Self:
The internal process of survival.

Stage 1   Daydreaming and Imaginary Friends

Stage 1 is the first level of unfolding and constitutes a mild reaction to a traumatic event. It creates a disturbance within self (loss, neglect, abandonment and/or rejection). The traumatic experience doesn't overwhelm all defenses but requires some distancing from reality. The boundary around self weakens making way for partial separation, yet the core remains intact. Such restructuring makes it possible to distance self from reality while altering thought and perception of the trauma. It is the act of achieving an altered mindset or state of altered consciousness that allows temporary disconnection from reality. An increase in episodes of daydreaming or the development of imaginary friends (Diagram 6) to avoid reality makes the phenomenon observable.

Daydreaming and creating imaginary friends are normal and healthy expressions of growth. Imagining is a child's way of adapting to life. Usually those behaviors stop as the person gets older, adjusts to fears, develops mental filters, and learns to cope with reality.   Sooner or later during development others will squash the practice and label it inappropriate. The message from other adults will be "grow up" and "stop living in your head".

The ability to perform both normal functions shows that the imagination is active and capable. Mature adults daydream daily. It is a device used to survive a boring meeting, an uncomfortable situation, or to pass time waiting for a plane. In adulthood these behaviors are referred to as "spacing out" or "just thinking." Daydreaming is a healthy practice if nurtured and appropriately used.

If daydreaming and imaginary friends are connected to the occurrence of a mild trauma, they will continue until the person arrives at a feeling of safety. Yet when such behaviors last beyond normal developmental periods and are directly tied to more traumatic events, they become the gateway to the unfolding continuum.

So just because you have kids who have imaginary friends or daydream, it doesn't mean that they have been traumatized or abused. But if there is a trauma and you see those characteristics present, it could be the first stage of the continuum.

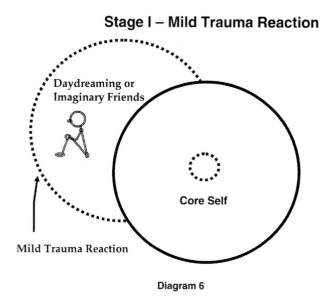

Diagram 6

Stage II Dissociative Reaction

Stage II is the most identifiable portion of the continuum. Travel to this stage is the result of a single traumatic event. If stage 1 was not strong enough to assist in separating from the pain of reality, stage II allows for complete though temporary mental disconnection. With trauma-produced feelings of being emotionally overwhelmed, no more defenses available, and the body feeling trapped, movement to stage II is accomplished. It's a pure act of protection by making what is real – unreal, seeming as if it never occurred. To accomplish the unfolding stage the mind, body, and spirit instinctively link up with imagination to create an alternative path for survival. After completing this stage, mind, body, and spirit sever connections so that traumatic physical and emotional pain happening to the body don't register in the mind.

To withstand intense emotional pain and save the whole, the head symbolically disconnects from the body (Diagram 7). It's a structural change performed so that physical pain isn't registered in the head. The change occurs when the whole is threatened to the point where the central core needs to be hidden.

I think of the core from a practical point of view as being like the motherboard of a computer. It determines how the computer will run and connects all parts to a central control. It contains the blueprint of who a person will be if she maintains a pattern of healthy growth. The core contains all the qualities that make a person, human.

More important, I look at survival of the core from a symbolic standpoint. It contains three attributes unique to humankind: the self, soul, and spirit. Symbolically self is immobile, incapable of moving under its own power. The soul is imaginative and can create what is needed. Spirit is symbolically free and moves without bounds. Under a threat to the whole, spirit comes and picks up self, while soul creates an open window through which spirit carries self to safety. The soul will remain at its post until spirit returns with self and the three are united again. The above is in fact a symbolic description that mirrors the dissociative experience.

To gain a better understanding of this stage of the unfolding process, consider the following:

1) The core is the fundamental part of the whole and must be protected at all costs. If the core were to be captured or damaged, the person wouldn't be able to return to wholeness. So when a trauma is perceived as invading the boundary of self, the core is hidden away within an altered structure.

2) For the core to be concealed, it must be released from its boundaries, which are relaxed in attaining the altered state of consciousness known as a *dissociative experience.* The core is then symbolically carried away to complete the process of restructuring. The mental system (head) and the physical system (body) separate and establish what I term a state of *duality* (Diagram 7). At that point a protective dissociative reaction has been achieved. From the outside the unfolding process gives an impression of weakness because the person's intense focus is directed inward but it is actually a demonstration of the inner power, intelligence, creativity, and strength of self.

For example, a child under the age of six is asleep in bed, and the door opens suddenly in the middle of the night. Awakened, she looks up and sees a figure standing in the doorway. Backlighting distorts the figure into a fuzzy monster, who enters the room and begins to do painful things to her. Physically trapped, what can the child do? She can't push the monster off, can't scream, and can barely breathe. She is overwhelmed, and has no working defenses available. The child feels as though she will die. Feelings of hopeless and helpless arise from her inability to fight off the attacker. Faced with no way of escape and no physical options, her imagination intervenes and takes on a new role. It helps her make reality unreal, mentally changing her molester's shape into a big furry monster (a reasonable and creative emotional response) enabling her to survive the experience through repression. The imagination unites mind, body, and spirit to save the whole. To protect self the child believes the event was a nightmare.

This second stage of unfolding shows the reality of an innate gift called *dissociation*, a state that almost all of us can attain if needed. It isn't an indication of being weak, immoral, bad, dirty, damaged, or defective. Rather, it is a demonstration of strength, intelligence, creativity, and power. Duality increases the area available for hiding the precious core.

Even though the unfolding is done out of love for self and preservation of the whole, splitting up the whole allows a conflictual relationship to develop between dissociative self and physical self. It is fostered by what is said during the trauma and creates intense self-judgment. Cognitive distortions, criticism, lies, vicious and degrading language are the tools a perpetrator uses to control a target. They turn the focus from the abuser's sick behavior to the victim being at fault. Over time their application results in self-phobia that tears down the victim's strength and strips away all emotions, self-worth, self-confidence, and self-esteem. The unconscious or conscious use of those tools bonds her with the perpetrator and insures loyalty to their secrets. The outcome is a total disowning or rejection of the body. The traumatized person no longer trusts her own feelings, judgments, or behaviors. Life becomes nothing more than an empty, numbing existence, trapped in a hated body.

On another level the dynamics of the relationship between physical self (body) and dissociative self (head) become that of mutual distrust. Both sides have issues of abandonment and rejection with each other. Physical self doesn't trust dissociative self because dissociative self abandoned physical self during the traumatic event. Dissociative self doesn't trust physical self because it is dirty or damaged by not stopping the event. If physical self and dissociative self cannot trust one another, they must look outside of themselves for personal validation, affection, attachment, direction, love, nurturing and control. The longer the conflict-ridden relationship continues after the original trauma, the harder it is for the parts to mend, accept, and forgive.

Such a relationship is complicated by the values, expectations, and distorted perceptions taught by the outside force. For instance, a child being sexually abused hears during the act, "I'm doing this because you are so beautiful and special, and it feels good to you." But in fact it's very painful. Sometimes the incongruence of pain vs. love creates a state of confusion in the mind that it distorts the truth. Should she believe the words of the abuser or the pain she's feeling? If the child doesn't like self, acceptance of the distorted values occurs. Right or wrong, from that point forward she thinks, acts, and feels as outside forces dictate. Extreme devotion develops with or without emotion (loyalty) to the "secret." Loyalty doesn't come from love for the perpetrator but because of the one-on-one intense, shared experience (the Stockholm Syndrome). As long as extreme devotion stays active, the secret will remain locked away.

As a result of the hiding of the core in stage II, dissociative self feels a loss of physical self and vice versa. Preservation and preparedness for the next invasive trauma or overwhelming loss becomes the major objective. Hypervigilant monitoring of the environment becomes a constant activity. During this stage a voice begins to form in the left side of the brain (see Abuser's Values, p 83). It is negative, controlling, critical, and oppositional to one's own internal voice. If the self-voice says something is good, the negative voice insists that it's bad. As self-trust decreases, the negative voice gains strength and control over thoughts, feelings, and behaviors through criticism, distortion of the truth, fear, lies, and threats.

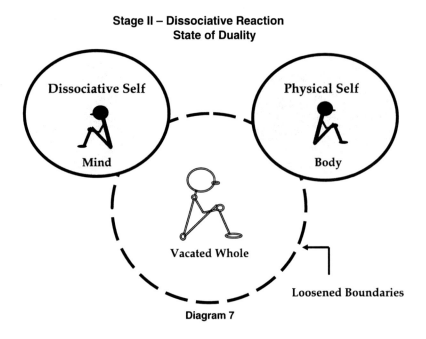

Diagram 7

Stage III Out of Body Experience

This is the act of completely disowning the body (Diagram 8). Survivors have reported, "From across a room I saw a little girl who was being hurt." or "I remember looking down on my body." Research into clinical death experiences show that people who returned from death reported "leaving their bodies" or "looking down on their bodies." If people are able to do so at death, there is a good chance they have the ability to do it when it's needed in life.

Advancing to this stage results from an increasing number of traumas, the elements of movement (degree of sensitivity, age at time of trauma, intensity, repetition, severity, and amount of pain) escalating when the previous stage was unable to hold back or stop the rising pain. The movement affords greater distance between dissociative self and the frequent pain physical self is going through. Structurally there is not much change from the last stage. A subtle shift on the continuum allows the abused a greater chance to disavow the emotional and physical damage happening to the body (Diagram 7). The person then experiences a feeling of being out-of-body. No longer does she feel that the body (physical self) is part of her. From that point on the body becomes estranged and is the focal point of the acquired self-phobia. Incidents of self-punishment start, reflecting the degree of hatred for the body. In stage III the person acquires the skill needed to objectify the body, thus eliminating any feelings of guilt about acts of self-punishment.

Addictive patterns begin to surface in stage 3 - such as alcohol and drug abuse, eating disorders, self-mutilation, obsessive-compulsive urges, and more. Addictions increase the ability to disown the body while punishing it at the same time. They are used mainly by survivors to medicate past buried traumatic pain or to achieve a state of numbness even at the risk of becoming addicted. An addiction isn't as frightening as all the unresolved emotions that have been hidden away. So to fight off more trauma and its associated pain, addictive patterns are linked to the dissociative reaction from the last stage to further isolate the pain from consciousness. The more skilled the person becomes with out of body experience, the more she can ignore and deny pain.

Stage III – Out of Body Experience

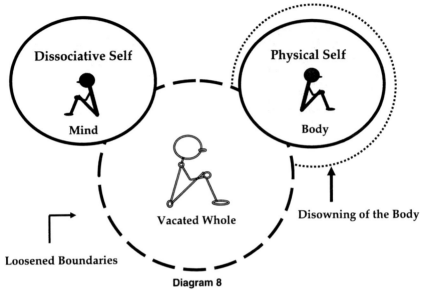

Diagram 8

Stage IV Compartmentalization Reaction

The inability to stop the more active elements of movement in the face of ever-present trauma weakens inner resources, and the victim unfolds higher up the continuum. Stage IV of unfolding is the symbolic process I term *compartmentalization,* and it is the next position on the continuum. It lays the groundwork for a structural shift from duality to multiplicity by constructing areas for storage and future movement because of fear that the weakened defenses will make the core more vulnerable to capture (Diagram 9). This stage is a defensive act that allows for the separating of the parts of the whole. A number of storage areas are creatively constructed and unfold off the outer perimeters of dissociative self and physical self. Compartmentalization occurs when both selves perceive that their boundaries aren't strong enough to protect the core making it vulnerable to further invasion (trauma). The construction of storage areas allows the victim to hide what is overtly or covertly forbidden. It safely stores away qualities and traits (intelligence, beauty, emotions, behaviors, feelings, functions, expressions, independence sexuality, spirituality, skills, talents, thoughts or truths) that are self-deemed forbidden. Displaying any of the above characteristics would result in more punishment.

Think of compartmentalization as the construction of a symbolic chest of drawers on each side of the victim. Both chests are tall and have many drawers. One holds the aspects associated with the mind and the other holds those associated with the body. Every time something is pointed out as unacceptable or forbidden, it is stored away in one of the drawers on the appropriate side. It is taken out of the drawer, used as needed, and replaced once its usefulness is over. The person is coconscious with each aspect.

For example, a child who is violated in her bedroom almost every night at 11:30, anticipates what will happen and experiences anger and fear. The door swings open, and there stands the perpetrator. She knows she's trapped and defenseless. The first thing the perpetrator sees on the child's face is anger. He looks straight into her eyes, points a finger, and says, "If I ever see that look again, I'll give you something to be angry about." Or "If I see that look on your face again, you'll wish you were dead." So what does the child do with her anger? She has a natural right to be mad, but she's learned that any display of anger brings more pain. She is convinced that the perpetrator will hurt her even more mentally and physically. So in order to survive, she accesses her imagination and creates a symbolic chest of drawers right there next to her. She symbolically puts her anger in one of the drawers and closes it. She's convinced that complying with the perpetrator's demands will reduce punishment and pain in the future. The child feels that if the pain doesn't increase, she's thinking, acting, or feeling correctly. It becomes distressfully clear that her choices, judgments, or decisions are always wrong. Hopelessness and helplessness strengthen with the realization that she should only think, act, and feel as she is told.

To expand the example, the same child is also viciously criticized for being stupid. She learns that smart is unacceptable, so she stores her normal intelligence in another drawer and she acts stupid or admits stupidity to please her abuser. And she is told repeatedly, "This is our secret; promise you will never tell." Truth goes into another drawer and the secret into yet another. The symbolic development enhances the little girl's ability to repress traumatic memory while increasing her distance from reality.

Compartmentalization provides the dissociative self and the physical self greater areas in which to hide the core and store the person's "normalcy" for later retrieval. An abused person uses the compartments as reference (advice) or tools (function). Depending on the need, the two selves use stored personality aspects together or individually to help the victim live in a dysfunctional environment. What is stored in the different compartments gains more importance each time it is accessed.

Things on the physical-self side are assigned identifying characteristics such as angry part, evil part, innocent part, intelligent part, etc. The dissociative self is assigned functions such as relationships, job duties, and education, etc. Labeling characteristics and functions is a way to navigate the maze of life. Each item in the compartments is a symbolic representation of the whole personality. But the original power and strength of the whole is diminished by being spread among the various compartments, thus weakening the person's overall ability to function.

Stage IV – Compartmentalization Reaction

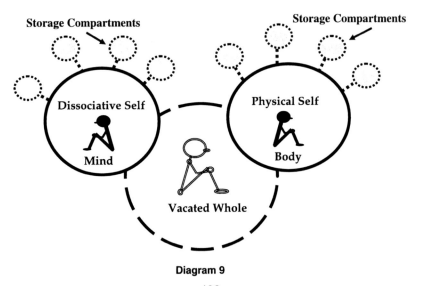

Diagram 9

Stage V Fragmentation Reaction

If the previous stages fail to stop the escalating episodes of trauma, emotional pain, and the other elements of movement, a person unfolds to the next stage, which I term *fragmentation*. It describes the act of investing more into saving various aspects of self and set up more of a maze to hide the core. Further distance is required from reality because of mounting pain. When compartmentalization fails to halt repeated onslaughts of trauma, dissociative self and physical self fortify the newly created storage areas boundaries and make the compartments ready to move into. The small circular extension's boundaries are solidified and made suitable for residence (Diagram 9). Solidification represents yet another attempt at preserving the whole, but in distinct, independent regions. Dissociative self and physical self can now more easily divide into smaller parts for greater safety and protection. Dissociative self and physical self vacate the state of duality (Diagram 7), subdivide (the process of dividing the parts into more parts) and take up residency in the solidified compartments (Diagram 10). Every new trauma is perceived as a deeper invasion and a weakening ability to hold off pain in the two previous areas (dissociative self and physical self).

In this position the fragments take on greater responsibility and independence. Even in a weakened state they play a strong role in the sufferer's functioning but co-consciousness remains. The fragments serve as her consultants. She is aware of all the stored fragments of self and relies on their participation to be able to operate in reality. Once the transition is complete, each fragment is assigned an identity, a function, and a voice enabling it to perform the consulting role and exert more influence. Fragmentation allows a person the ability to interact with reality in an altered state from a safer distance. At this stage, mastery of dissociative skills is of utmost importance, and more time is spent in dissociative episodes, making less time available for daily activities.

Stage V – Fragmentation Reaction

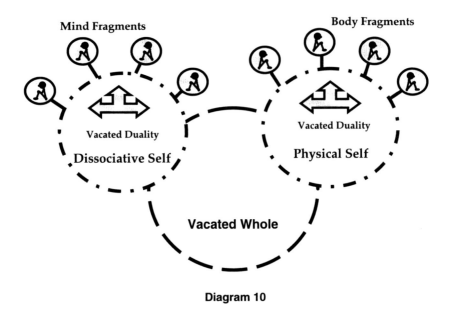

Diagram 10

Stage VI   Multiplicity Reaction

Stage VI is at the far end of the continuum, where a person crosses a line into what I term *multiplicity reaction* (formerly know as Multiple Personality Disorder, MPD and now Dissociative Identity Disorder, DID). Attaining stage VI is only necessary if the victim has experienced maximum levels of all six elements of movement, including sexual and physical abuse before the age of seven. When physical and emotional pain becomes intolerably severe and frequent, previously formed defenses are no longer effective. This stage represents the act of disavowing coconsciousness and recognition of complete reality. Awareness of all the traumatic events is impossible and at this level unbearable. Amnesic barriers are erected to stop cross contamination. They don't permit any information or memory flow between fragments. Division between dissociative self and physical self deepens, and complete disengagement from the Stage II structure takes place (Diagram 11). The book *Sybil* and its 1977 movie rendition tell an excellent story that accurately describes stage VI.

In stage VI a fragment from the last stage is transformed into what is generally termed an *alter*. It is also described as an *ego state, altered personality*, or *regressed state*. Since I believe that the term *alter* carries negative, destructive connotations of separate personalities living within a damaged person, I prefer to call it a *symbolic aspect of self*. The ability to develop a symbolic aspect of self or alter is a wondrous and innovative thing. Collectively the sum of all the fragments equals whole self and symbolically remains connected to the original structure.

The symbolic aspect of self is a finely developed defense mechanism that allows for the highest degree of protection. An alter is given complete independence, its own identity, function, and voice along with other unique characteristics. An alter is assigned a specific function and develops in relation to the traumas it experiences and the amount of time spent in reality. Fear, anxiety, and impending dread make up the predominant atmosphere in the new system of parts. Transformation occurs when the fragmentation structure loses power and lacks sufficient stability to resist constant pain.

Characteristics of the Symbolic Aspects of Self

Symbolic aspects of self have well-defined characteristics. Although the fragments may appear to be very different, all stem from within a single human being.

Each symbolic aspect of self has

1) its own life and its own independent way of relating, perceiving, thinking about, and remembering life.

2) an amnesiac barrier separating it from the others to stop any leakage of pain, memories, loyalties, or secrets.

3) its own memory bank for just its interactions with reality.

4) only one purpose, and that is survival.

5) a duty to protect the whole.

6) its own method of numbing that accounts for the multiple addictions found in this stage.

7) its own system of self-punishment.

8) its own abuser's values (negative voice) received during time spent in reality.

9) its own secrets and threats.

10) its own physical characteristics, voice inflections, health problems, body image, and dress.

11) its own perception of self and life at a specific age.

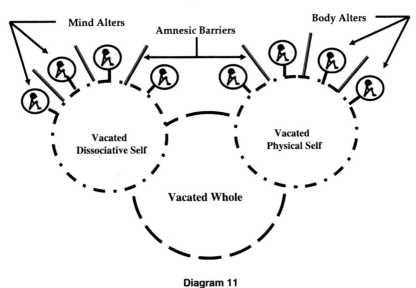

Diagram 11

Stage VII

There is one more possible stage of unfolding that can happen. This is a rare form that results from the person being exposed to ritual or cult abuse (Diagram 12). Certain clandestine groups use acts of torture, isolation, mutilation, starvation, imprisonment, violence, mind-altering drugs, brainwashing, and vicious language as part of their rites or traditional practices to control followers. Such abuse puts a child's self preservation system to the maximum test, causing rapid unfolding from multiplicity to severe multiplicity, creating minor outgrowth from a major alter.

Let's look at an illustration using the major alter whose function is anger. Because the anger is not strong enough to handle repetitive brutal attacks, further defense is needed. To compensate, the major anger alter unfolds into two minor alters: rage and violence. They assist the major alter in protecting the system.

Stage VII – Severe Multiplicity Reaction

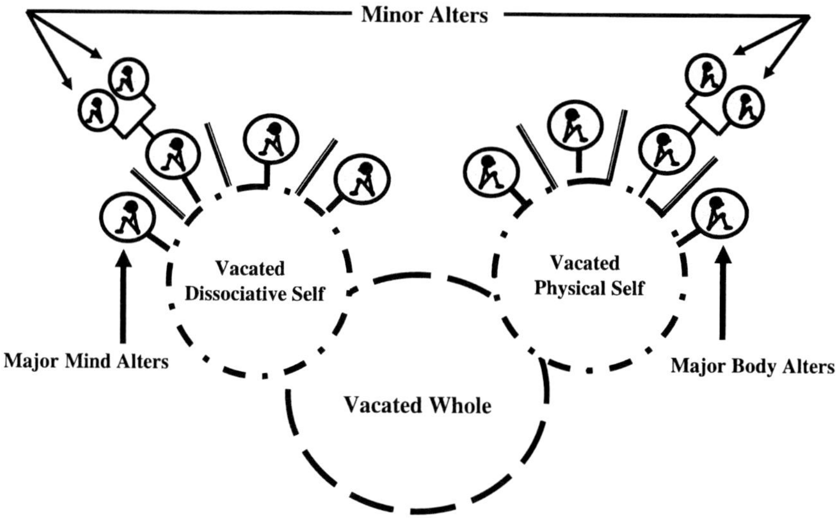

Diagram 12

I hope that discussing the seven stages of the continuum has increased your awareness of the unfolding process of self as a creative gift. Its stages reveal the extent self will go to in order to survive the same traumas that kill many children every day. The unfolding of self is an incredible process when performed by an adult (Stages I-V), but it's miraculous when performed by a child younger than seven (Stages I-VII).

Summary

Unfolding is a proactive act of defense against trauma accompanied by a decision to survive. It is clear that the process isn't an act of defectiveness. It demonstrates, rather, what it takes to maneuver up each stage of the continuum - strength, intelligence, creativity, and power. Survivors are unjustly labeled as weak, dangerous, damaged, or broken. Unfolding is a healthy adjustment to a sick event, not a negative manifestation of deep seated disease. General ignorance of how surviving trauma works causes survivors to be pigeonholed as abnormal, sick, insane, or violent.

I have sought to show you that there is hope for recovery. Where is it to be found? The answer is in the original process itself. The survival process was symbolic, yet the resulting symptoms were treated by traditional methods. The helping profession focused on the symptoms and dismissed the symbolic progression of surviving. So if unfolding is a symbolic survival route, then the same symbolic ingredients can assist in developing a recovery route. Indeed health can be found in a symbolic reversal to a state of wholeness.

Chapter 7

Recovery

The answer to recovery doesn't lie in memory retrieval or analysis of the past traumatic event. The saying "nothing is more confusing than the past, and there is nothing more cleansing than the future" really stuck in my head. What if all the inner resources, symbolic elements, and strategies used by a human being to survive could be understood, reversed, and applied using a positive technique to facilitate recovery? I never found relief or recovery from analyzing, reviewing, or interpreting my trauma memories. The more I delved into my past, the more I needed to numb out or escape. The encounters with that same material just seemed to retraumatize me. I noticed relief only came when I unknowingly ceased to focus on the past and focused on a specific goal such as school or some other project.

My initial work started on the aforementioned hypothesis. Could a safe and protective technique be designed to help a person return self to whole? Once I understood the stages and the specific elements that caused further unfolding, my awareness opened a new mode of thinking. The survival process as I see it occurs clearly on a symbolic basis; therefore the recovery process should also be based on symbolic theories, skills, and techniques. I envisioned a procedure that would use the power, strength, and creativity of symbolism to mimic the original journey in reverse. At that point I seemed to be released from the shadows and entered the light of awareness. Like most survivors I attempted recovery with preconceived negative attitudes and ideas about recovery and *nothing wished for ever came true*. Recovery worked for others but not for me. My preconceived notions severely limited the results and insured failure. Everything I learned showed me that trauma recovery is a process – not a happening, stroke of luck, particular medication, or scientific method. There isn't one procedure that works universally.

Besides the mechanics of the process, other issues must be addressed, and that's how survivors interact with the idea of recovery. People have directed them how to think, act, and feel for so long that they don't know any other way to be. Others told them they would never get better or do things the right way. An aftereffect of trauma is that the survivors become self-defeating, feeling they don't deserve to recover because of what they were taught. Many wish for recovery but mentally find the concept foreign and confusing. Sometimes survivors ask for what they don't really want, believing in their hearts they won't get it. That paradox reflects their incongruent thinking about recovery. If by chance survivors ever make it into recovery, some unconsciously end up rejecting it because it feels unfamiliar, or not the way they imagined it should. They reject the very thing they seek – success. Survivors lack the skills to participate in recovery because their skill acquisition had focused on ways to survive rather than become.

Yes, recovery feels uncomfortable, undeserved and impossible, yet recovery is about being honest, nurturing, and supportive to self. I found in my work with survivors that they don't want to reveal their defects or flaws to others and especially to self. It would be more healing to view survival as an accomplishment or the ability to unfold by invoking a miracle, but they end up focusing on emptiness, hopelessness, and perceived damage.

Survivors think bad things just happen to them, and misfortune was always their fault. No matter how much they did for others, it was never enough. Their good deeds were never returned in kind. No matter how much effort they put into filling their emptiness by accumulating relationships, objects, money, and status, it never worked. What they learned was that answers weren't found outside of themselves but inside.

I think the following issues profoundly influenced my recovery from trauma. They weren't necessarily the only ones or the correct ones, but they were obvious during my effort to recover. For recovery to be successful, understanding how a trauma survivor thinks and the issues that result from that thinking are as important as the mechanics of the process itself.

Mind-sets

An essential lesson here is that humans are what they think. People can only think, act, and feel as they were taught - nothing more. If someone is taught positive things, then the thinking tends toward the positive. Conversely the thinking can tend toward the negative. So the person's mind-set is an extremely important factor in the success or failure of their recovery.

Mind-set is here defined as an inflexible mental attitude, rigid thinking, or a fixed state of mind. It determines how a person will feel, act or think about a specific subject. I truly believe that recovery is 50 percent attitude and 50 percent skill acquisition. So mindset is pivotal to a person's willingness and ability to work for recovery. Mindsets can develop on different levels: physical, mental, emotional, or spiritual. There are three types which are pertinent to this population (1) victim (2) survivor and (3) recoverer.

The following descriptions refer to states of mind and not to labels or processes. People attempting to resolve psychological trauma get stuck in such states of mind without being conscious of them. Hopefully an awareness of these will help them move forward.

1. Victim Mind-set

A recurring thought that permeates this state is "everything happens to me." Characteristically, a person with this type of inflexible thinking remains connected to the past and views past events as foreboding templates for future scenarios. The person lives life in a hopeless and helpless state of mind, constantly waiting for the other shoe to drop. She thinks "If I do nothing, I won't get hurt." With little or no trust in other people or in self, she isolates and withdraws from society, hoping to avoid contaminating other people with her bad luck. This state of mind is an externally oriented mode of thinking. Personal validation is sought only from others. All thinking, feeling and behavior are based on negative messages.

This type of mind set refuses to disconnect mentally from past traumas, hurt, and pain. The sufferer denies or ignores flashbacks, hoping the dire events never actually happened. With years of practice she cultivated skills to develop a proficiency at being a victim. As a result her mind-set becomes a way of life and for some, a personal status. Someone with a victim's mind-set focuses on and lives in the past, thus having no present or future. She thinks recovery isn't obtainable because of her unworthiness. If recovery actually happens, it must be by mistake or through a stroke of luck.

Summary of the Victim Mind-set.

- Emotions are "numbed out"

- Behaviors are that of acting helplessness, hopelessness, and depressed.

- Speech is "I give up." or "It doesn't matter."

- Objective is to increase victim skills.

- Management of this mind-set is to unconsciously seek traumatic triggers and situations in order to get better at being a victim.

2. Survivor Mind-set

I warmly refer to this state of mind as the "warrior." The person's attitude is a mix of anger, bravery, and fear. The recurring thought that permeates this second mind-set is, I just survived that event. I won't let anything or anybody hurt me again. I will win over trauma at any cost. Examples: I just survived –going to the mall, having sex, a job interview, a meeting at work, etc. Anyone with a survivor's mind-set views everyday life as an endurance test. The warrior continues to fight battles of past traumas in the present, this is so consuming they neither live in the present or plan for a future. Since life is an ongoing battle, the warrior is always on guard, waiting for the next engagement. Her objective is to win that next fight, loss, or trauma, all the while accumulating new weapons to use in the next battle. Someone with this mind-set approaches life with anger, rage, and a deep need for vengeance. A warrior thinks recovery has to be a long, hard trial, so someone or something outside her has to force self into recovery.

Summary of the Victim Mind-set:

- Emotions are anger, rage, revenge and rigid; feels "forced upon."

- Behaviors are that of acting combative, aggressive, resistive, and guarded.

- Speech is "Nothing will beat me again," or "I face my fears and conquer them."

- Objective is to get through the current battle and move on to the next.

- Management of this mind-set is to be consciously hypervigilant with arms at the ready like a good warrior.

3. **Recoverer Mind-set**

This one is different in that it is initiated by conscious decision, not past events. The recurring thought is, I don't know if I really want to _____ (event or situation). Let me experience it first, and then I will make up my mind to do it again or not. The attitude is a mix of confidence, control, and faith. Such thinking is a far cry from the two previous mindsets. A recoverer accepts that life is an assortment of learning experiences. She views the future with fear but follows through on decisions anyway. Precious time isn't spent on predicting or judging but on experiences of the moment. Past events are "hold" lessons, used as references to assist functioning in the present and making plans for the future. She understands that the future is unpredictable and that falling down or having setbacks is a part of life's experiences. If a setback occurs, a recoverer picks self up and nurtures self with plenty of TLC. Personal value comes from self validation, not from outside. This person views life with awe and excitement. Life is seen as a challenge not a chore or burden. Taking responsibility, being able to respond appropriately, and keeping self's word for decisions made form the new attitude. The recoverer is willing to accept the consequences for what self does. A person with a recoverer's mindset doesn't define self in terms of performance. She stops seeing events as success or failure, right or wrong, good or evil but as lessons learned. Patterns for future behavior are based on those lessons and become the foundation of the future. A recoverer understands that the journey of recovery from trauma is fluid and will have its ups and downs. Validation is confirmed from within self.

Summary of the Recoverer Mindset.

- Emotions are experienced as they happen without judgment and doubt.

- Behavior is to face life proactively as a challenge, not as a chore or burden.

- Speech is, "Nothing will beat me again" or "I face my fears and conquer them."

- The objective is to increase lessons learned through experience.

- Management of this mind-set is building on a foundation of experience to increase life skills and plan for the future. It's important to understand that moving back and forth between all three mind-sets is common. As attitudes and personal strength fluctuate, the person changes her mode of thinking, though some do get stuck in one mind-set. How fast she recognizes and resets self's attitude is the measure of success in recovery.

Characteristics of a Recoverer

- Experiences the present and references the past but doesn't relive it or dwell on it to enhance the present.

- Sets plans for the future while making the best of today with acquired tools.

- Experiences each life event individually before deciding if it's beneficial or not based on whether it takes self toward or away from recovery.

- Doesn't attune to abuser's values (negative mental tapes) but daily recites positive affirmations to reprogram thinking.

- Accepts and forgives the core self no matter what.

- Feels life, learns from it, grows at own pace, and lives the best way self can.

- Enters into recovery based on self-decisions (I will get better!) and seeks help when needed without shame or self-judgment.

Summary of Mind-sets

Victim and Survivor Mind-set		Recoverer Mind-set
(Rejection of experiential input)	or	(Acceptance of experiential input)
Familiarity	or	Risk and decisions
Reactive	or	Proactive
Defenses tools	or	New tools for creativity
Loyalty to abuser	or	Loyalty to self first
Old behavior patterns	or	New behavior patterns
Fear, panic, anxiety, shame and guilty thinking	or	Positive Thinking
Judgment, punishment, and sabotage	or	Faith, proactiveness and nurturing

Critical Issues of Recovery

There are two issues that can severely influence a person's ability to begin or stop movement in recovery. Professionals in different disciplines working with people who have experienced trauma are well served to understand the power and threatening force that these topics present in the therapeutic environment. No one attempting to recover from trauma is free of these dangers.

The first issue is the abuser's values and the second is loyalty. If a recoverer (survivor actively working on trauma recovery program) isn't aware of both, recovery is generally sabotaged; and the person won't understand why self isn't succeeding.

Abuser's Values

During a traumatic experience a victim may go into an active dissociative state (an altered state of consciousness). While in that state any sound, statement, or voice is recorded in the mind of the victim.

Noise is an everyday part of life, but constant and painful sounds from the past are not supposed to be. Daily auditory input can shape attitudes and perceptions and influence how someone thinks, acts, or feels. Hearing trauma sounds is a common experience reported by survivors. They can be a simple noise (a car crashing, wood snapping, howling winds), a voice (words spoken during the trauma experience) or a mix of confusing and frightening sound. Trauma sounds always feel intimidating, critical, commanding, and/or controlling.

Repressed traumatic sounds return to consciousness in the form of audio flashbacks. They may not reach a person's conscious awareness for some time after the trauma, perhaps not for years. Once the audio flashbacks begin to play in a person's head, however, they create fear and confusion. Victims have described them as creepy, critical, demanding, demeaning, frightening, intimidating, negative, scary, shaming, shocking, threatening, triggering, controlling, or commanding. Audio flashbacks shape the survivor, influencing the person's thoughts actions and emotions from that point on. With the passage of years fatigue and repeated submission to this auditory barrage causes greater devotion to secrets.

The voices/sounds referred to as *Auditory Flashbacks* occur inside the survivor's head and are experienced as real. They are not the auditory hallucinations known as *psychotic voices*. Even though produced in the mind *psychotic voices* are experienced as coming from an outside source. *Audio flashbacks* are experienced inside the head in exactly the same form they were recorded.

Audio flashbacks are what I term *abuser's values*. They are defined as a sound, noise or words recorded in the brain while mental filters were down because of an altered state of consciousness. *Abuser's values* are re-experienced audio recordings of the sounds from a trauma. They can function independently from visual flashbacks or work in conjunction with them. When they take the form of commanding comments they make the victim fearful, guarded, hypersensitive, skittish, and emotionally over reactive to sounds coming from their environment as well as those emanating from within their own heads. Abuser's values playing over a period of years can cause the person to disdain, disown, hate, severely judge and reject self. They create what I term self-phobia, an extreme sense of hatred for self.

Understanding the concept of abuser values and its effects is crucial to the recovery process. Even the sanest people have negative and critical thoughts about self. Such thoughts are common, healthy, and unavoidable in the fast-paced, performance-oriented world in which we live. In healthy people they stay just that – thoughts - and are never turned into self destructive behavior. But abuser's values are more destructive, intense, threatening, and troubling than normal critical thinking. Obeying abuser's values results in self-destructive behavior toward self. Accepting the commands of abuser values increases loyalty to the secrets, thus asserting more control over the person.

Cognitive distortions, criticisms, and viciously degrading language are some of the programming tools perpetrators use to influence and control their victims. They are the means by which they turn the focus away from their own sick behavior and direct it toward tearing down the victim's confidence, emotions, worth, judgment and esteem. Using them the abuser can objectify the victim, thereby avoiding any sense of guilt for hurting another person. The process seems to sanction the perpetrator's own behavior in much the same fashion that a terrorist's intense anger justifies his lawless acts of violence.

When abuser values are spoken words they are a collection of programmed negative thoughts made up of unattainable expectations, cognitive distortions, distorted values and degrading language addressed to the victim. After continuous exposure to their replay, the abuser's values become the standard for how the person will think, feel, behave, relate, interact, and interpret self, including intelligence, body image, and perception of reality.

Identifying or diagnosing abuser's values is difficult because they become tightly intertwined with the victim's daily perceptions and thoughts about self and the world. Pervasive thoughts such as I hate and distrust myself; I have a dark side I don't like; I'll never amount to anything; I'm someone that no one will ever love because I am so damaged; or I can't succeed in anything, are common statements heard in the minds of trauma victims.

One way to understand abuser's values is to say that all people see themselves through binoculars. If the binoculars are properly positioned and focused, they will see themselves as whole, valued, complete, competent, and acceptable. Unfortunately, not everyone has excellent binoculars and knows how to use them. As a result of trauma the victim might be looking through the wrong end of the binoculars. They can still see through them, but everything is distorted from reality. Additionally, the lenses may be smudged with external cognitive distortions, criticisms, vicious and degrading perceptions. In that view self is seen as small and distant, incomplete, defective, insignificant, different, hopeless, and powerless. This distorted view or false image of self causes a strong emotional reaction that develops into an aversion to and rejection of self, which mirrors self-hate but is so intense it causes a complete self-phobia.

Once the abuser's values are installed, the mind controls the person rather than the person controlling the mind. They trap the self in a negative, fearful, secretive, dark world. Self is totally cut off from reality, and the victim is unable to have an emotional relationship with self, other people, or the world.

Victims don't have to exist in the state I just described. They can make a decision to stop reacting to/or obeying the abuser's value commands or statements. Self has the power to regain control of mind and use it as a tool for recovery.

Loyalty

Loyalty is a normal, learned value taught every child and is defined as the quality of being extremely devoted, unswerving in allegiance, and faithful to a cause, ideal, custom, institution, or product. It has been viewed throughout history as a cherished quality that is needed for family cohesion. Loyalty is the glue that keeps units together. It's a characteristic admired and highly valued in American society.

For anyone who has survived an abusive upbringing, dysfunctional home, or a trauma, the issue of loyalty becomes distorted. These experiences cause a victim to perceive life as an all or nothing proposition. Extreme opposites form in the person's mind representing light (love & nurturing) and darkness (hurt & pain). The abused person thinks in black or white. From that point on she perceives life events and other people as good or bad, righteous or evil, loyal or disloyal, right or wrong. Closeness and relationships become dangerous and illegal. From then on there is no gray area, no middle ground.

Telling secrets is considered to constitute a breakdown of loyalty, the ultimate act of betrayal. Within a family structure, disclosure to anyone, even another family member, is an act of treason punishable by exile or death. Other retaliatory acts can take the form of being dismissed, disowned, or even tortured mentally or physically. At the time of the first trauma the core identity fragments for internal protection and preservation of life. Once that happens, the victim accepts stated threats and becomes devoted to the distorted abuser values. Whether the threat to the secret is fact or is meant to intensify fear or is used as a method of control, it is real in the mind of the abused.

Betrayal by the perpetrator is never considered, but if his prey even thinks of disclosing the secret abuse that act is viewed as the ultimate betrayal. It is an unforgivable breach. Betrayal is an act punishable by the abuser or by the victim's own self. It may take the form of addictive relapse, self- mutilation, or other dangerous behaviors.

It's widely accepted in the healing professions that the first step toward recovery is exposure of the "secret." Yet in actual practice, within hours or even minutes of disclosure, the scariest barrier – loyalty - rears its ugly head. Overwhelming feelings of being wrong, betrayal, and immanent death surface and result in a strong need to retract the disclosure. Common statements heard by victims who have revealed painful secrets are: "I made it up," or "It was a lie; please let me take it back," or "It was a creation of my imagination." The person's total energy instantly focuses on protecting both the secret and the perpetrator at any cost. The victim would rather reinstate her excruciating symptoms than continue to betray the abuser and face death. Any act that serves loyalty to the secret, even against self, is necessary and legitimate.

Thus loyalty, a normal and respected value, can cause severe alienation from self, significant others, family, therapists, and people in general. It most certainly can halt recovery. So while working with a victim's loyalty requires constant effort and monitoring, it is the key to their growth and successful recovery.

Recovery Isn't

I have discussed in story form and through description what I believe a human goes through internally in response to traumatic experience and its ensuing aftereffects. I talked about the root of the unfolding process, the theory, how it developed, the stages, the resulting symptoms, aftereffects, symbolic connections, mind-sets, loyalty, how thinking has to change to reverse it, and the basic principles of recovery. Now I would like to make clear what recovery isn't.

Recovery isn't about waiting for it. It doesn't knock at the door. Hiding from the past by ignoring, denying, withdrawing or isolating self won't make the pain go away. Symbolically burying one's head in the sand won't keep the abused hidden from the horrors within. All spare time and energy is spent trying to keep past secrets suppressed and traumatic experiences from intruding into the mind or disturbing everyday life.

Recovery isn't something that happens automatically. It has to be to put into operation. It is the act of taking back what was taken away - regaining power over thought, feeling, and behavior when the odds seem hopeless. It means changing acquired negative or frightening beliefs about getting well. Recovery is as much a proactive process as the survival process was when it went into action. It's creating and adopting a positive, empowering belief about recovery, facing real fears and starting new behaviors anyway.

Recovery isn't owed as payment for experiencing trauma and time served in its effects. You can sit around feeling entitled, but nothing will happen.

Recovery isn't time consuming. It doesn't have a beginning or an end. The hardest lesson to learn about recovery is that it's an ongoing experience. It is a discipline that must eventually become an accepted way of life.

Recovery isn't a literal process but a symbolic one. If the loss happens symbolically and is invisible to the outside world, then recovery is also internal and invisible. The answers to resolution are not found or validated from the outside, they lie within. Recovery starts with looking inside and doing what was never allowed – accept, forgive, like, love and attune to self. There is no magic pill which takes away the terrible mental images, physical hurt or emotional pain.

Recovery is not revenge on the perpetrators, the event, or self. It's about developing a relationship with every aspect of self and thereby mending the original relationship that was broken so long ago. It isn't looking back and finding the mistake that caused bad things to happen. There wasn't one! Nor is it a question of getting rid of aspects of self perceived as bad or evil. The person may not be happy with what she had to do to survive, but good or bad, all parts make up the whole. Feelings of resentment serve no useful purpose. Recovery means taking the risk to learn about the power and strength that exists inside. Remember that the brain can only produce what it is taught. The wonderful thing is that the brain can relearn and begin to understand what health is.

Commitment to the process is of utmost importance. Recovery is earned by following through on promises no matter what happens. It means believing the work being done in the present will flourish in the future. Recovery is earned by taking back control of thoughts, feelings, and behaviors without excuses.

Recovery isn't indecisive. The first step away from the effects of trauma is making the decision to recover and that may be the hardest part of the process. Someone else has always made the decisions. Don't be reactive, make the first move and decide. Know that once the decision is made there's no turning back. If a promise is made to self and broken, the consequences can be worse than the original trauma.

Recovery isn't losing the memory. It's about gaining awareness that self did not cause the trauma, it just happened. An outside force stole the light of life and shrouded it in darkness. Memory wants to be recognized, not analyzed or re-experienced.

Recovery isn't ignorance. Being released from not knowing is accomplished through learning, education, and experience. Additional knowledge helps in examining the truth of old forced beliefs, perceptions, and values. New formation can store right on top of the old. When an event happens, the new formations give more options on how to think, feel, and act. The more that's learned, the more options there are to choose from and the less fear is experienced. Fresh knowledge creates ideas, internal power, creativity, imagination, and strength. It also allows freedom from lies, fears and controls of the past. Once awareness is raised, ignorance can no longer be invoked.

Recovery isn't an easy process, but neither is living in darkness and terror. At first reinstating a good relationship with self is hard and painful. Things will be learned about self that the victim didn't want to know. But new and wonderful things about self will also come to light. It's necessary to stay in contact with present reality to learn that the past happened but is not happening now.
Recovery isn't without sacrifices. By changing, everything self had may be lost. Whatever was used to numb pain will no longer work. There are no guarantees in recovery.

What is recovery? It's growth through creating and implementing sets of new thoughts, emotions, behaviors, values, expectations, boundaries, definitions, and affirmations. It's being human, imperfect. It's healing and taking back what was wrested away by force. Recovery is acceptance and forgiveness of self. It's a risk. Changing is a risk; life itself is a risk.

Yes, recovery is possible. It can be one of the most enriching and fulfilling experiences of a lifetime. If the self was able to unfold in order to survive, it can refold in order to grow.

Developing Friendship with Self

Making the decision to enter recovery and committing to the process is just the first step. The next one can be more frightening. A question always preceded making the decision. Now that I've made the decision to accept and forgive myself, how do I have a relationship with myself? I would like to share some thoughts on that idea. Self is instinctively hidden because of a desire for safety. Once a connection with self is restored, it should be embraced, loved, and nurtured, not ignored, judged, abandoned, or rejected. Healing is the process of recovery and means establishing a relationship with self to fill the unfamiliar emptiness and increase the feeling of wholeness (being in balance) to become what people are meant to be.

Traumatization robs a child of the time for healthy personality development and maturation, so an authentic relationship with self never forms. As an adult, such a relationship feels awkward, confusing, illegal, and forbidden. It was learned that having a relationship with self was wrong. Being in a relationship and doing what that other person wanted was the way to success, even at the cost of a relationship with self.

So how are skills acquired to attain a fulfilling, deep, satisfying, and meaningful relationship with self? Here are some building blocks that assist in the process. Though each building block is only a guide, together they form a foundation for a friendship based on listening, communicating, caring, committing, honoring, honesty, responsibility, rewarding, risking, and trusting. Without a strong foundation true friendship can't develop with self. Other friendships will be unsuccessful as well. There are no automatic friendships or guarantees that any relationship will last forever. Developing a relationship takes hard work, investment, loyalty, and consistency. To be successful, the following need to be worked on.

1. **Frequency**. The first building block might seem just common sense, but it's a place to start. Authentic friendship grows naturally when time is spent with self. The more frequent the contacts in a relationship the deeper the connection. Meaningful and frequent contacts with self must be a priority.

2. **Authenticity**. The biggest fear about attachment is exposure to rejection, abandonment, and pain; so a relationship mask is worn. Involvement is faked by controlling the situation or directing other people. Fooling others may be attainable, but fooling self is impossible. In recovery circles the saying is "You are only as sick as your secrets." Be willing to share hidden secrets with self. Authenticity is about experiencing and revealing all feelings honestly to

self. That allows a budding relationship and the beginning of healing. Be open and truthful with self. Be real.

3. **Support.** The world is self-defeating enough without further assistance. Self-defeating attitudes and thinking only make a person feel more alone. If a relationship with self is desired, self needs encouragement, and understanding - to be listened to and to have feelings validated. Be sensitive to all feelings, stand up and honor them. An internal friendship derives its strength from self-support; so the more support self receives, the stronger it grows. Self can't be what the Creator intended without being balanced, and that requires a strong footing in order to achieve equilibrium. With self there is everything; without self there is only emptiness. Self-denial, self-anger, or self-disowning breeds weakness in a friendship. Accept and uphold all the wonderful characteristics, abilities, and talents self brings into being. To achieve growth all systems need to be working in harmony. Be your own cheerleader in life!

4. **Respect.** It's all right to admire differences and acknowledge self even when there is dissatisfaction with performance. Respect is an act of having a special regard for someone without criticizing or judging. Everyone has many thoughts, feelings, and behaviors that frustrate and annoy. Complaining, denying, or ignoring "faults" won't resolve issues or bring you into a closer relationship with self. Judging and criticism contain nothing positive. Don't make perfection or absolute compliance with expectations a basis for friendship. Demonstrate some old-fashioned respect and show self how much worth it has. Give self undivided attention, learning what it wants. Ask for clarification if something is misunderstood and listen without interrupting. Respect isn't automatic; it's earned even with self. Over time respect builds a balanced, better, stronger, and more authentic relationship with self.

5. **Acceptance.** Next to fear, judgment and perceived rejection destroy relationships more quickly than anything else. Not being accepted feels like rejection without cause. In the past self was judged to be unacceptable, so even as we would act with another person, we shouldn't act like we are more important, better than, or in control of self. Rather, receive self willingly without standards or expectations. Mutual acceptance is an important element in any relationship. Be willing to recognize different characteristics and qualities of self that might have gone unnoticed. Be open enough to admit wrong or misunderstanding. Judgment projects the air of being a know-it-all. Be willing to say, "I need your help," or "I was wrong," and "forgive me." If those words cannot be uttered to self, the foundation will crumble.

6. **Openness.** It's sad when you attempt to hide the truth from self. Truthful and open answers are a mark of authentic friendship. Being open and being connected go hand in hand. Good feedback without lies is needed to navigate through life. Don't live in relationship darkness any longer. Connect with all the great talents, qualities, and unique characteristics hidden within self. Openness to self will produce growth. Healthy friendships allow frustration, sadness, and even anger to be expressed. Disagreement and conflict are healthy if handled appropriately and within boundaries.

7. **Forgiveness.** The world isn't a perfect place. Hurt and pain are normal in relationships. Friendship is imperfect, which means you are certain to get hurt sometimes even in a strong relationship. The issue isn't the hurt itself; but how it is handled determines whether a friendship deteriorates or improves. Forgiveness and trust are major building blocks. Forgiveness is a willful act done in a short time. Since it is an act of kindness and giving, resentment must be put aside. Trust means assured

reliance on character, ability, strength, or truth and is built slowly over time. Trust is earned when deed and word are consistently reliable. There is no genuine friendship without forgiveness because grievances will arise. Be willing to risk.

8. **Boundaries.** Friendships are risky when you have no idea how to think or act. Constructing a boundary is the act of setting limits agreed upon within the friendship. All of us have the right to define friendship and to determine our own values, expectations, lifestyle, and priorities. Boundaries allow self to function within fixed limits, adding predictability, safety, and protection. Don't leave self without the comfort of knowing what is expected.

9. **Confidentiality.** "Loose lips sink relationships" is appropriate for what not to do with this building block. Close relationships never develop without confidentiality backed by strongly agreed upon boundaries. It is confidentiality that increases and assures safety within friendships. The quickest way to destroy any relationship is overstepping boundaries and letting out confidential information. If confidentiality of shared information is an agreed upon boundary that information needs to stay within the relationship.

10. **Loyalty** – Here is the last and most important building block. The preceding blocks are good, but loyalty is at the apex of any friendship's structure. It is defined as an *act of extreme devotion, unswerving in allegiance.* Loyalty isn't automatic but requires a decision and a commitment. Allegiance is a necessary ingredient in achieving a solid relationship with self. Friendships grow when there is loyalty and a unity of purpose.

Understand that the formation of a friendship is not based on sameness. Using the ten building blocks doesn't mean that each person involved has to act, look, think, or feel exactly like another to be an authentic friend. Use the blocks as a guide. Individuality can foster a healthy friendship, and there can be unity without uniformity.

If these ten building blocks are applied and practiced, they will help in the formation if an authentic friendship with self.

Chapter 8

Incorporation Therapy

Research has proven that survivors of trauma have difficulty responding to traditional types of therapy. Traditional methods tend to be literal and concrete and thus create confusion. Many survivors actually end up feeling invalidated and misunderstood and relapse into destructive behavior patterns such as addictions, self-mutilation, self-sabotage, and/or reacting to triggering elements of traumatic memories. Members of this population tend to become retraumatized whenever they do any therapeutic memory work, and as a result PTSD symptoms intensify. The literalness of traditional methods fails to address the symbolic nature of the survival experience as a response to trauma.

This chapter describes a safe symbolic methodology designed to facilitate stabilization of posttraumatic stress disorder symptoms. I call it *Incorporation Therapy*. It is a unifying process offering assistance by way of a refolding back to a symbolic state of wholeness (balance) that opens the door to recovery. Incorporation Therapy provides a way to help survivors in reconfiguring their internal structure on a symbolic level that mirrors the unfolding process. It isn't meant to be a cure, It is a way to go back down the continuum to symbolic wholeness. It's a safe and protective procedure that allows symbolic taking back of what was lost during the traumatic experiences. Reconfiguration helps all psychological, physical, and spiritual systems return to a state of wholeness.

During a traumatic event the mind can automatically encapsulate traumatic memory, breaking it down into emotional, and physical components. The emotional component is composed of two elements – pleasure and pain. The physical component contains the elements of pleasure and pain along with what the survivor saw, touched, smelled, and heard.

Therapeutically, the emotional component is the more difficult to resolve. Emotions remembered always surface in the consciousness before actual memory of the physical component does. The repressed emotional component emerges with the same intensity as when it was first experienced. The natural reaction is to shut down the latent emotion or numb out the pain before overwhelmingly hurtful emotions re-traumatize. Though there may have been years between the traumatic event and the present, without the acquisition of new coping skills remembering the emotional component overpowers the survivor and throws her into reliving the traumatic experience. The associated emotions are equal to or more intense than the original ones and give rise to feeling trapped, anxious, and terrorized. Such devastating feelings inhibit the ability to stay in the present, protect self, and function normally. The person becomes emotionally reactive and defensive. Acting out, denial, rationalization, relapses into addiction, self-mutilation, and other numbing-out behaviors are the result of reliving traumatic experiences. The victim becomes even more critical and negative toward self for its inability to protect. All that is left is a sensation of emptiness or loss of self.

Faced with memory encapsulation the emotional component absorbs whatever was too painful to deal with at the time. What I have found is that the buried emotional component turns out to be more frightening than the memory of the act and forms a barrier to resolution.

Incorporation Therapy is designed to provide a safe, and protective proactive method for dealing with the emotional component from a revisiting position. It allows for protective distance from the emotional component while providing a secure environment in which to rescue self. This symbolic method gives the survivor the opportunity to rescue the core (self) without having to live through the pain locked in the emotional component. Once self is rescued from the memory, the memory is altered (restructured) from that point on. The emotional component is dissipated, and the memory no longer poses a threat.

Six Characteristics of Unfolding Self

The process of the unfolding of self as a response to a trauma requires the cooperation of many different personal characteristics. From beginning to end the process is internal and symbolic in nature. The more I studied this miraculous process, the more it made sense to identify and decipher its properties. If the characteristics of the original act were found, then maybe the same characteristics in different configuration would facilitate development of a method to assist in re-folding.

I discovered six characteristics that work together on a symbolic level to complete the survival process (unfolding). These were:

1. Imagination
2. Dissociative State
3. Self
4. Soul
5. Spirit
6. Symbolism

1. *Imagination* is an underrated function of the brain and is seen as being synonymous with child's play. But it plays a significant and unique role, serving many functions in the survival process when self is faced with trauma. It dreams, creates, alters, and imagines worlds that are safe and protection that reality doesn't offer. Imagination is a powerful tool that appears to be the mechanism by which the mind can make what is real, unreal. It can create anything and because it has no bounds, everything is possible to it. The imagination works in conjunction with the other five characteristics to assure survival. When not under traumatic conditions, the imagination serves as a communication bridge between the conscious and unconscious mind. Its operation and use of symbols can be observed in dreams.

2.   The *dissociative state of mind* is akin to daydreaming, but magnified fourfold. It allows one to escape mentally and blocks an unbearably painful reality. The altered state of consciousness can be as simple as consciously disconnecting from a boring speaker at a workshop. It seems to serve symbolically as the path on which to travel up the continuum.

The *core* is the foundation of one's being. It contains three elements innate in everyone – self, soul, and spirit (discussed in three, four and five). The core blueprints for all that a person is. If the core is damaged or lost, self cannot be what it was intended to be. The core is instinctively protected and saved at all costs.

3.   *Self* is the first element of the core. It holds characteristics that belong uniquely to oneself and serves symbolically as the self's connection to reality. Self can be viewed as the self-esteem element of the core.

4.   *Soul* is the second element of a person's core and has been described as its most imaginative element. The soul is one's connection with the imagination and one's own depth. The soul is the part of the core that believes anything is possible, and anything can be imagined, even surviving trauma. It operates on faith, believing strongly in what can't be seen, touched, or felt. The soul serves symbolically as the architect and builder of whatever must be constructed mentally to allow the unfolding. Soul can be viewed as the self-worth element of the core.

5.   *Spirit* is the cores third element. It can be seen as the life-giving force, essence, or the connection with the Deity. The spirit is the essence of a human being – her energy, and freedom. This function can be viewed as belief in God, higher power, or what one perceives as a "power greater than self." It serves symbolically as the vehicle on which the core moves along the continuum. Spirit is viewed as the core's self-control element.

6. *Symbolism* is the last of the six elements used in the unfolding of self. It serves as the language that all the characteristics use to communicate during the process.

Incorporation Therapy Technique

Without a stabilization method a person can't truly focus on recovery without years of hard work. My objective was to design a method to shorten that time frame. Incorporation Therapy assists in the stabilization of a person's internal structure. Its main mission is to relieve and reduce the intensity of PTSD symptoms. Simply said, it helps the refolding process.

Alteration of the symbolic internal structure after exposure to trauma is so complex and extensive that there had to be two procedures created to deal with it. The first addresses the acute portion (duality) of the continuum, and the second type concentrates on the severe end (multiplicity). These two types are based on the same symbolic language and all six characteristics, but are configured much differently. The severe end of the continuum requires far more structure and boundaries than does the acute.

Two other important criteria are considered in the designs.

1. Incorporation Therapy is survivor driven so that the patient has a sense of empowerment and control. In comparison hypnosis is practitioner driven. I want a person to be in control of reversing the process just as she was when the original process took place. To a survivor, control equates with safety.

2. Incorporation Therapy was designed so that the patient can free herself from the procedure at anytime. All she has to do is open her eyes and the procedure stops with no side effects. Further, the entire method is approached as a revisiting method, not one that causes re-experiencing of painful events.

Platform Method

The platform method of Incorporation Therapy is for individuals who have undergone acute traumatic episodes and loss of self. The traumatic experience could be the death of a significant other, divorce, status loss, catastrophic disasters, domestic violence, robbery, rape, neglect, torture, abandonment, confinement, or abuse during which the individual unfolded up to the fourth stage of the continuum.

Although given from the patient's viewpoint, the first part of this book, Barb's Story, gives a clinically accurate presentation of the platform method of incorporation.

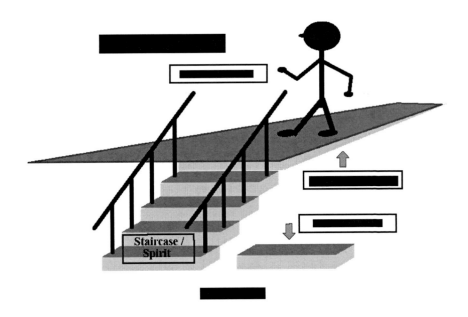

All six characteristics are combined in the construction of the platform and staircase. The platform serves as a foundation, and the staircase acts as the means for movement. To accomplish this task the patient has to access her imagination. That offers an entry point into the storage area where traumatic memories are kept. Refolding occurs with movement down the stairs and then up again. The main objective is to rescue the self that was hidden and then forgotten long ago. Using the platform method allows the patient to revisit a memory, view it safely, enter it and rescue self without reliving the experience. When the self in the memory is symbolically removed to safety, the emotional component evaporates, and the memory becomes merely a picture without associated emotional content.

Dome Type

The multiplicity end needs a greater degree of structure and boundaries because the original foundation had been stretched so far in order to distance self further from the reality of severe, repetitive trauma episodes and losses. But movement up the continuum to stage seven over taxes and distorts the foundation.

Diagram 15 shows the increased structure and boundaries using the same six characteristics. An orderly gathering of the system of alters under the protection of the dome releases the emotional component and breaks down the amnesic barriers that separate alters. The ending structure symbolizes wholeness. Remember, wholeness is not a cure or an end to the journey. It is just the beginning of another recovery.

Dome Type

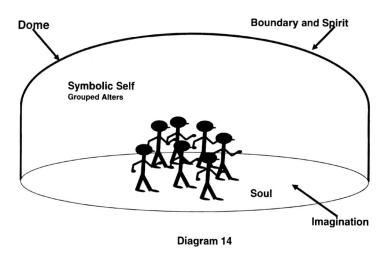

Diagram 14

If the platform or dome method is successfully used, it reduces the feeling of emptiness, stabilizes the internal chaos, and lessons the intensity of the emotional component, and the constant focus on validation turns into growth.

Chapter 9

Steps Toward Recovery

1. Make the choice

    Make a decision for health.

    Decide not to stay in pain any more.

    Commit to each decision.

    Choose to help self first, not to fix events of the past.

2. Gain awareness

    Decide to understand properly the mechanics of what has happened.

    Learn about the effects of trauma from appropriate resources.

    Seek help from experienced professionals and appropriate support groups.

3. Take responsibility

    Take back control of thoughts, feelings, and behavior.

    Responsibility means keeping promises to self no matter what.

Stand up and face the consequences and rewards for decisions made.

Honor the new direction you set for yourself.

4. Accept and forgive self

Accept aspects of self back into yourself without judgment.

Forgive self and not the perpetrator or the event.

5. Develop a relationship with self

Communicate, negotiate, and compromise with self regularly.

Nurture, support, and love self.

Follow through with promises and commitments made to self.

Do what you say you'll do for self.

Take a risk on new behaviors.

Be a friend to self.

6. Identify desired changes

All people have the right to change anything in self they want to as long as it does not hurt self or anyone else.

Create the self you want to be.

Realistically design and write down how you want to think, act, and feel.

7. Take action

> Practice and practice until the new thoughts, actions and feelings become second nature.

> You don't have to believe it; just practice.

8. Don't Give Up on Yourself

> Do not turn your back or give up on self.

> Don't judge your every move.

> If you have a setback pick self up and go back to the Third Step.

Remember, you are worth the hard work!

Epilogue

In closing I'd like to share the survivor's credo that offers a guiding principle to live by during recovery. It summarizes all the ideas, theories, and principles I have discussed in this book. If repeated often it can serve to direct, empower, energize, focus and inspire.

Survivor's Credo

Guide me to reach beyond my old fears

and perceived limitations.

Assist me to regain control of my thoughts,

acts, and emotions.

Support me in taking back my power from

those who put limitations on me.

Grant me the strength to take credit for

my decisions, responsibilities,

and consequences.

I am!

Bibliography

Allen, J. (1995). *Coping with Trauma: A Guide to Self Understanding, p 14*

Andriani, C. (2004) *Shock: The Aftermath of Trauma*, Enlightened Choices, Vol. 7, Issue 1, Melbourne Beach, FL, p 1

Giller, E., president and director, The Sidran Foundation: http://www.sidran.org/whatistrauma.html

Carnes, Patrick J. (1997). *The Betrayal Bond: Breaking Free of Exploitive Relationships*, Health Communications, Inc., Deerfield Beach, FL p Xvii, 5, 8, 26

Briham, D.D. (1994). *Imagery for Getting Well: Clinical Applications of Behavioral Medicine.* W.W. Norton & Company, Inc., New York – London

Friesen, James G. (1991). *Uncovering the Mysteries of MPD* Here's Life Publishers, Inc. San Bernardino California.

Herman, J.L. (1992). *Trauma and Recovery: The aftermath of violence from domestic abuse to political terror,* HarperCollins Publisher, New York, NY, p 1,2,33,34,96,135,154, 173-195

Jung, C.G. (1964). *Man and his Symbols.* Aldus Books. London.

Marshall, R., M.D. ABCNews.com/Oct2001 Report

Ross, C.A. (1994). *The Osiris Complex; Case Studies in Multiple Personality Disorders.* University of Toronto Press. London.

Salter A.C. (1995). *Transforming Trauma: A Guide to Understanding and Treating Adult Survivors of Childhood Sexual Abuse.* Sage. Thousand Oaks, CA:

Sargant, W. (1997). *Battle for the Mind: A Physiology of Conversion and Brainwashing.* Malor Books, Cambridge, Mass.

Schwarz, R.A. (1995). "Separating Fact from Fiction on the "False Memory" Question." *Innovations in Clinical Practice: A Source Book* (Vol. 14) Professional Resource Press.

Steinberg, M. and Schall, M. (2001) *Stranger in the Mirror: Dissociation the Hidden Epidemic.* Cliff Street Books. New York. p 3, 11, 16.

Tollefson, W.B. (1993). "The Forbidden Betrayal: Loyalty within Sexual Trauma." *Treatment Center:* Feb. Issue.

Tollefson, W. B. (1994). "Secret Shame: Effects of Severe Repetitive Trauma." Inner Values, Inc., Melbourne Beach, Fla.

Tolin, D.F., Montgomery, R.W., Klienknecht, R.A., and Lohr J. M. (1995). "An Evaluation of Eye Movement Desensitization and Reprocessing (EMDR)." *Innovations In Clinical Practice:* A Source Book (Vol 14). Professional Resource Press.

Whitfield, CL (1995c). *Memory and Abuse: Remembering and Healing the Effects of Trauma.* Health Communications. Deerfield Beach, Fla.